Dogs in Health

Dogs in Health Care

Pioneering Animal-Human Partnerships

JILL LENK SCHILP

DOGS IN OUR WORLD
Series Editor Brian Patrick Duggan

McFarland & Company, Inc., Publishers
Jefferson, North Carolina

LIBRARY OF CONGRESS CATALOGUING-IN-PUBLICATION DATA

Library of Congress Cataloging-in-Publication Data
Names: Schilp, Jill Lenk, 1947– author. | Duggan, Brian Patrick, 1953–
    editor.
Title: Dogs in health care : pioneering animal-human partnerships / Jill
    Lenk Schilp.
Description: Jefferson, North Carolina : McFarland & Company, Inc.,
    Publishers, 2019 | Series: Dogs in our world | Includes bibliographical
    references and index.
Identifiers: LCCN 2019034757 | ISBN 9781476673943 (paperback : acid
    free paper) ∞) | ISBN 9781476636962 (ebook)
Subjects: LCSH: Dogs—Therapeutic use—History.
Classification: LCC RM931.D63 S35 2019 | DDC 615.8/5158—dc23
LC record available at https://lccn.loc.gov/2019034757

BRITISH LIBRARY CATALOGUING DATA ARE AVAILABLE

ISBN (print) 978-1-4766-7394-3
ISBN (ebook) 978-1-4766-3696-2

Front cover images: Labrador Retriever therapy dog © 2019 Shutterstock;
inset Red Cross dog collar, Berlin, Germany, 1914–1918 (Science Museum,
London)

Printed in the United States of America

McFarland & Company, Inc., Publishers
    Box 611, Jefferson, North Carolina 28640
        www.mcfarlandpub.com

To the Dogs
Dolly, Chloe, Pine Cone, Nuggett,
Dante, Max, and Junior

Table of Contents

Acknowledgments

Two of my middle school teachers once told me, "You should be a writer." It took a long time for me to believe that was possible. It turned out it was. I took the long road to get there. Many people helped me along the journey. I am grateful to each of them for guiding me in their own way.

Decades ago, two librarians in Clifton, New Jersey, showed a young girl how to find the best dog books on the shelves of a cozy library on cold, lonely New Jersey days. It was on those shelves I discovered the magic of dogs. I learned the power of a good dog story. I traveled with Buck in Jack London's *Call of the Wild* and consumed dog books until the seed of the dog writing dream sprouted.

I am grateful to my high school science teacher who was the first to show me the rewards of telling a good dog story. I was a senior in high school, and a paper was due. I confessed the truth to my teacher. I had not completed the assignment because my dog Chloe, a nearly perfect black dog in every way, had just the night before devoured my Biology book. Anticipating some professorial skepticism, I then produced what remained of the demolished book. I told the "dog versus book" story in vivid detail with props. I set the scene of the crime and gave a rich, if not entirely accurate, characterization of the ordinarily docile Chloe who I claimed, "must just like Biology." I explained the missing bookbinding and why pages 50–200 had those teeth marks and were now just shreds. I spared no adverb. I became convinced that my first true dog story must have been compelling because I got an A on the term paper and for the rest of the school term, my teacher greeted me with a snicker and asked. "How's your dog doing?" At graduation, that same teacher wrote a three-word message in my yearbook, "To the Dogs." Thus began my appreciation for the power of nonfiction. I was on my way to telling dog stories.

I am grateful to the Dog Writers Association of America (DWAA) who first recognized my work with the Maxwell Award for my blog. That gave me the confidence to tackle a book project. DWAA led me to Brian Patrick Duggan, the editor of the Dogs in Our World series at McFarland. I thank Brian and McFarland for providing the opportunity and support to tell the stories of the Dog Pioneers of health care.

Susan Schultz, Carolyn Marr, and their dogs Dolly and Bevo were my inspiration, teachers, mentors, and role models in animal-assisted therapy and showed me what it means to be a pioneer. I am grateful to them for allowing me to share their stories. I also thank the Monday Fun writing group in Richardson, Texas, who are my best cheerleaders; they inspired me and challenged me with writing prompts, serious Scrabble games and the friendship of storytellers.

Thank you to Steve Fontenot and Dr. Tatia Fontenot and Bellin for sharing their story with me and to the Seeing Eye Inc., the International Association of Human-Animal Interaction Organizations Pet Partners, and the Freud Museum in London for allowing me to use material and photos. I am grateful for Cynthia Orticio for her assistance in preparing the manuscript.

Writing a book takes patience, confidence, endurance, resilience, and a sense of humor. My mother, Norma Lenk, showed me by her courageous example never to give up and never to quit. She also showed me that just about everything in life can make you laugh. I thought about that when my printer kept interrupting me to tell me it wanted more paper.

I am grateful to have learned from many dogs in my life—Dollie, Chloe, Pine Cone, Nuggett, Max, Dante and Junior. From the dogs of my childhood to Junior who sits next to me today, my canine family taught me and showed me their stories and my own. I heard their voices as I wrote the chapters of this book. They were the first to show me first-hand the enduring power of the human-animal bond.

I owe a debt of gratitude to the many rescue dogs that have passed through my life. They showed me the redemptive power of love, that you can create your own second acts, and that the right dog will always find you.

Finally, my husband, George, provided the things that make my writing dreams possible. I am grateful to him for understanding when I gave him "that look" when he interrupted me at the keyboard while I was busy telling dog stories. He kept me and the printer running throughout this project. I am grateful for the privilege of living my life with a best friend who tells me, *"nobody will ever love you as much as I do … except the dog."*

I am a lucky woman.

Pioneer:
One who goes before to open the way for others to follow

Preface

I grew up believing that a girl and her dog could change the world. For the next 30 years, I worked in nursing and health care improvement. As a health care professional, I was always interested in learning about innovative men and women throughout history who found creative and better ways to care for people. In all those years, I never stopped believing in dogs and their magic. Along the way, I discovered something else. I was right about dogs changing the world.

In roles from medic to muse to modern medicine, our canine partners inspired humans to improve health care in unusual places and unexpected ways. Throughout history dog pioneers have shown humans what can be learned from canines about comfort and healing. But we had to be paying attention.

This book is about the change that occurred when dogs and humans worked together and learned from each other how to transform health care and each other. It is about the science, art, and often the poetry of the human-animal bond. The book also explores what we may owe our canine partners in return for their service and devotion.

I had been thinking about dog pioneers for years. As a young girl I had discovered the power of a good dog story. Growing up, I spent most of my summers and after school hours at our one-room community public library in New Jersey, where I searched for and found the dogs whose adventures filled my days and my dreams. Later in my life, James Herriot's series of books, especially *All Creatures Great and Small* and *James Herriot's Dog Stories*, inspired my quest to learn more about how dogs and people help each other and the human-animal bond.

As I went on to study nursing in undergraduate and graduate school, I discovered pioneering dogs along the way. I found Jofi the chow beside the couch of psychiatrist Sigmund Freud. I learned about Cap, the sheepdog who visited Florence Nightingale's dreams, and I discovered a dog named Jingles

1

who raced child psychiatrist Boris Levinson to answer a knock on the door to his office. I read the story of the sled dog heroes who delivered the life-saving vaccine in a diphtheria epidemic. I saw how each dog uniquely was a pioneer in health care. Later in my health care career, I was impressed with the evolving human partnerships with dogs that I saw emerging in a variety of modern health care settings.

I was finally inspired to write about the dog pioneers by my dog Junior and my own transformational experience of the human-animal bond. A few years ago, as I began my retirement from a full-time health care career, I became a registered therapy dog team with Junior, a golden retriever. Junior and I visited a variety of health care settings. Junior was a registered reading education assistance dog, so we also read with children in libraries as part of our therapy dog work. The children we read with were often struggling with learning to read and were reluctant to read aloud. Reading was not much fun for them until Junior arrived and plopped down on his monogrammed blanket with a supply of dog-themed, dog-eared books and his wagging tail.

During our reading sessions, I noticed that Junior was a terrific listener. When children sat down to read to him, they seemed to know that they had someone interested in them. It did not matter how well they read. At a reading session, Junior's body relaxed as soon as he entered the library. Once I placed his red fleece blanket in a corner on the floor, I gave the "down–stay" command and Junior remained there until the 45-minute session was up. He might curl up in a tucked half circle. He often shut his eyes. Sometimes he rolled over to allow the reader to rub his soft golden retriever belly.

When Junior and I read with a struggling reader, I had fun and so did the young reader. Together we traveled on a journey through an imagined world. As I joined in the magic of these reading sessions between young reader and canine, I rediscovered the joy of reading with someone. I watched Junior. The dog's nonverbal communication and the reading were soothing to all three of us: the reader, the dog, and me. I wondered: *Is Junior having a great time too?* I hoped so.

Junior wagged his tail as the child's voice changed the tone and the dog edged closer to rest his head on the child's lap when the child would look up at him. I usually joked with the young reader that Junior might give away the ending of any book we read because he always wagged his tail when he knew the "good guys" were going to win. I suspected that Junior sensed that reading time was different from his other activities. I thought that Junior probably just enjoyed the petting and all the attention, but the young reader and I often decided together that Junior enjoyed the story and already knew the ending.

In our reading sessions, I discovered that reading with each other connected us, that the quality of the reading was not as important as the gift of the time together. I saw a way to connect. I saw how Junior did it. I felt it. The reader, the dog, and I did not need words. We listened. We understood. I realized that, if we watched, listened, and tried to understand, there were lessons in communication and connection our dogs might teach us.

I had lingering questions: Why do people react to dogs in the way they do? Why do we learn from dogs things that we cannot learn on our own? Why are dog stories so compelling? Do therapy dogs enjoy their work? I decided to turn to the dogs themselves to find answers.

The stories of these pioneering dogs span decades, from the trenches of World War I to the bed of a critically ill child in a modern intensive care unit—across periods of social change and innovations in health care. It was a time when humans' relationship with dogs was evolving, and we were beginning to recognize dogs as sentient beings rather than tools. We were starting to see what dogs, as our partners, could contribute to health care, often in unexpected ways.

Primary and secondary sources for the chapters and information about the dogs and their human mentors included interviews, books, letters, scientific journals, professional societies and organizations, websites, and archives. Several books were particularly helpful in providing historical information about the human mentors and their dogs. Hilda Doolittle's *Tribute to Freud* provided a firsthand narrative of a patient's experience of Freud's chow Jofi's role in Freud's consulting room. Mark Bostridge's comprehensive biography *Florence Nightingale: The Making of an Icon* provided insight into the complexity of Nightingale and the provenance of the story of her dog Cap. Florence Nightingale's classic treatise *Notes on Nursing* provided details of nursing and health care reform and Nightingale's view on the value of pets in health care. Gay and Laney Salisbury's *The Cruelest Miles: The Heroic Story of Dogs and Men in a Race Against an Epidemic* provided not only a great read but also a vivid chronicle of the adventure of the serum run and a robust source for details of the race of sled dog heroes Togo and Balto. Leonhard Seppala's biography by his colleague Elizabeth Ricker, *Seppala: Alaska Sled Dog Driver*, written in 1930, provided background details about Leonhard Seppala, Togo, and the serum run. Morris Frank's memoir, *The First Lady of the Seeing Eye,* provided a firsthand account of German shepherd Buddy and Frank's journey as the first seeing eye dog team in America. Rebecca Frankel's book *War Dogs: Tales of Heroism, History, and Love* provided information about military dogs, and the *U.S. Army Medical Department Journal* April-June 2012 issue dedicated to canine-assisted therapy in military medicine was rich with details about animal-assisted therapy, the roles of Boe and Budge, and the therapy dogs' experience in the military. Finally, Dr. Aubrey Fine's *Handbook on Animal-Assisted Therapy: Foundations and Guidelines for Animal-Assisted Interventions* and Dr. Cynthia Chandler's *Animal-Assisted Therapy in Counseling* provided valuable information on the history, concepts, and practice of animal-assisted therapy.

While many excellent books have described the contributions of dogs to humans in broader contexts, this book focuses exclusively on transformative canine pioneers at the intersection of human health care and the human-animal bond. The focus of this book is the dogs' contribution to health care. It is not intended to be a comprehensive history of health care milestones, a complete biography of the human mentors, or an all-inclusive discussion of animal-assisted interventions. I have provided suggestions in the chapters for readers who wish to pursue these topics further.

This book is written for anyone interested in dogs, history, humane education, and the human-animal bond. It will also appeal to those interested in health care improvement and innovation and the intersection of animals and human health care.

An introduction to the book provides the principal themes, conceptual framework, and theoretical foundations for the healing aspect of the human-animal bond and a brief profile of each of the dog pioneers of health care and their roles in helping humans change health care. Nine chapters follow. The first eight chapters tell the story of a pioneer dog or dogs and explain their contribution to an evolving health care process. The chapters explore how these contributions influenced human understanding of the mutuality of the human-animal bond and how that knowledge and experience influenced health care.

In Chapter 1, the Mercy Dogs of World War I pioneer battlefield triage and rescue. In Chapter 2, Jofi, Sigmund Freud's beloved chow, inspires and teaches the father of psychoanalysis. In Chapter 3, an injured sheepdog named Cap becomes Florence Nightingale's first patient and part of the heroic narrative of Florence Nightingale, the founder of modern nursing. In Chapter 4, two rival sled dogs, Togo and Balto, each with their own talents, lead sled dog teams on a serum run to Nome to deliver desperately needed diphtheria antitoxin during a disease outbreak.

Buddy, a female German shepherd, pioneers a new frontier of independence for people who are visually impaired in Chapter 5 by becoming the first Seeing Eye dog in the United States. American psychologist Boris Levinson's dog Jingles steps into the doctor's consulting room in Chapter 6 to become a pioneering child psychotherapy cotherapist. Jingles inspires a classic book. In Chapter 7, Sergeants Boe and Budge, two Labrador retrievers, train to serve in Iraq to introduce a new stress reduction approach for U.S. troops.

Chapter 8 follows the trajectory of how animal-assisted interventions have become integrated into mainstream health care. Chapter 8 also explores progress in the search for a scientific base for animal-assisted intervention as a new generation of therapy dogs integrates the healing of the human-animal bond into mainstream health care. Animal-assisted intervention is explored as both art and science. Chapter 8 also examines the question: What is the difference between a service dog and a therapy dog? The names we call dogs involved in animal-assisted interventions are often confused. A definition of terms is provided in Chapter 8.

Chapter 9 concludes with a summary of the dog pioneers' contributions and a review of the common threads and challenges they faced. This chapter looks to the future of dogs' contribution and the humane implications of what we owe them in return. Chapter 9 also addresses our connections with other species and the implications of our shared world. An epilogue includes a note on my own experiences in the transformative nature of the human-animal bond. A glossary defines the medical and animal-assisted therapy terms used in the book.

I have presented stories about each dog to begin most chapters. These are my illustrations and interpretations of events based on research and sources that described historical events. I have made every effort to stay true to the facts or descriptions I discovered in the various source materials that inspired the stories. I was able to learn a considerable amount of information about the breed, lineage, and appearance of some, but not all, of the dogs. When details were not provided, I described the dogs based on their breed characteristics.

I believe our words and terminology matter in how we tell dogs' stories. Our language should recognize animals as living beings, not objects. I have attempted to use terms that represent dogs as fellow species who share our common world and to avoid stereotyping them with human-centered terms. I have avoided terminology that refers to dogs as tools, entertainers, or objects. I have described the dogs by gender (he or she, him or her) rather than calling them "it" since "it" implies an object. If the gender of the dog was unknown (as with Jingles), I used the masculine "him." If the animal's name was known, I have used his or her name. I have used the term *guardian, handler, or mentor* to refer to the human in the human-animal bond rather than *owner* to reflect human-canine partnership rather than an object relationship. In places where I have referred to *our* dogs, the use of "our" is intended to imply partnership (as in "our partners"), not ownership. I have avoided using the term *master* unless I quoted a primary source that used that term. Humans share a common world with dogs, and we are both parts of the animal world. Throughout this book, the term *animal* is used to designate only nonhuman animals but recognizes that humans are part of the animal kingdom and we share that common identity.

You may be familiar with many of these dogs' stories and may meet some of the dog pioneers for the first time. Whether you have read their stories before by other writers or this is your first introduction to their stories,

I hope this book will be the first to show you the dog pioneers' intersection with human health care and their unique contribution. I hope the book will inspire curiosity about your own experience with dogs and how dogs can change our thinking.

Finally, this book is not *just* about dogs. It's about human-animal collaboration and partnership and how the human-animal bond propelled health care processes forward. It is the story of the arc of the human-canine connections that changed health care. It's about the science and the poetry of the human-animal bond and the possibilities that occur when dogs and humans reach out to each other and find the healing potential of the human-animal connection.

I still believe dogs can change our world. We owe it to them to understand them and tell their stories. These are some of those stories.

Introduction

Human-animal bond:
A mutually beneficial and dynamic relationship between people and animals that is influenced by behaviors essential to the health and well-being of both.[1]

Dogs showed humans how to care for each other. That sounds like a big job for dogs. How did they do it?

Humans watched dogs, we learned, and together we changed the world of health care. As humans discovered the healing and teaching potential of dogs, our partnership with canines evolved and our view of what was possible expanded.

Most of us who enjoy life with a companion dog have probably been tempted to claim that Rover or Fluffy is crazy about us. We can tell by the way they look at us, even when we are not holding a double cheeseburger.[2] There now may be science to prove it.

In a 2015 study published in the journal *Science*,[3] researchers found that when dogs gaze into their special human's eyes, and the human gazes back, an increased concentration of the hormone oxytocin is produced and exchanged between the human and dog. The researchers found that the more the dogs and humans gazed at each other, the more oxytocin was exchanged. Oxytocin is essential in familial bonding and promotes feelings of attachment. It plays an essential role in social bonding and bonding between mothers and infants and has a role in socialization and stress relief. Results of the 2015 study showed that humans might feel affection for dogs similar to what they feel for family members and that human-like gazes in dogs brought rewarding effects for dogs and deepened interspecies bonding.[4]

Throughout history, people have both reaped the benefits of this unquestioned devotion and attachment and struggled to understand it. The incredibly strong bond that exists between humans and dogs creates the dog's willingness and dedication to serving us in roles from a Mercy Dog on the battlefield to a gentle therapy dog at the bedside of a critically ill child.

The Dog Pioneers of health care used their remarkable bond with us to show humans new possibilities in the processes of triage, public health practice, adult and child psychotherapy, and therapeutic communication. They provided symbols for our patriotism, metaphors for our most profound thoughts and fears, and companionship and comfort at the end of life. Our canine companions showed us how to listen, reduce our stress, and reduce the stigma of talking about mental health issues and how to heal our physical and psychological wounds.

Dogs changed health care in roles from medic to muse to modern therapy dogs and became symbols and metaphors for health care improvement. They transformed health care processes and opened new ways of thinking about triage and medical transport on the battlefield, mental health, psychotherapy, public health, nursing, independence for the blind, and the untapped possibilities of human-animal collaboration in modern health care.

The Dog Pioneers of health care and their work spanned decades—from the trenches of World War I to the intensive care unit of a modern-day hospital. Dog Pioneers served in World War I, helped a man who was blind brave the busy streets of New York in the 1950s, created changes in psychotherapy in the era of the Beatles and Woodstock, deployed in the Iraq War, and walked the halls of the modern hospital with their own business cards in the age of Facebook and Twitter. Along the way, humans learned more about dogs and each other.

Although our dogs were showing us their ability to heal and comfort, humans were not always paying attention. The story of the Dog Pioneers that inspired new ways of thinking about health care delivery has a long arc of unexpected human discovery about dogs' nature, their lessons for us, and our relationship with them as partners rather than as children, objects, or tools.

Just who were these Dog Pioneers?

Red Cross Dogs, also called Mercy Dogs, were trained to be first responders on the battlefield in World War I and became part of the process of a new art of triage, the initial sorting of wounded soldiers on the battlefield. Thousands of Red Cross dogs were used in World War I. It is likely more soldiers might have died on the battlefield had it not been for the search, rescue, and triage work of the Red Cross dogs. The Mercy Dogs not only helped with rapid triage and evacuation procedures, but they also represented a symbol of patriotism and sacrifice.

Jofi and Jingles, the dogs of psychotherapists Sigmund Freud and Boris Levinson, inspired change in psychotherapy. Both dogs decided to join the doctors in their consultation rooms and changed Freud's and Levinson's perspective of treating patients. Watching their dogs interact with their patients,

Freud and Levinson observed that dogs could have a calming effect on people and help humans identify and express feelings and fears.

Jofi, Sigmund Freud's chow, inspired the father of psychoanalysis to better understand his patients. Jofi opened the door of Freud's office, claimed her place under the famous analysis couch, and legitimized the unheard of concept of a canine cotherapist in the therapy room. Years later, Jingles, psychologist Boris Levinson's dog, would leverage Jofi's contribution by walking into a new therapy room to launch animal-assisted child psychiatry. Jingles so inspired Levinson that the psychologist later dedicated his classic book, *Pet-Oriented Child Psychotherapy*, to Jingles. Written in 1969, Levinson's book was the first to document the techniques of using animals in psychotherapy. Although his psychologist colleagues initially ridiculed him for his ideas on the benefits of pets, inspired by Jingles, Levinson continued to pursue his work, and his book still stands as a classic reference in animal-assisted therapy.

Dogs can serve as symbols that evoke feelings and mobilize energy for change. In Alaska's 1924–1925 diphtheria epidemic, Togo and Balto, along with other dogsled mushers and their dogs, were portrayed as heroes in newspapers across the United States as they successfully completed a dogsled run to transport badly needed serum to Nome. This dramatic transport by two rival sled dogs provided publicity that spurred an inoculation campaign that dramatically reduced the threat of the disease. The serum race spurred development of air routes that could provide better and more efficient medical supply movement and increased awareness of preventive immunizations.

Events with dogs can take on other symbolic possibilities. As a child, Florence Nightingale encountered an injured dog named Cap who became her first patient. Cap became a part of the vast heroic narrative of the Lady with the Lamp. Later, Nightingale reported mystical dreams that she had a mission to heal others. Nightingale's implementation of new concepts in infection control, self-care, therapeutic communication, and public health advocacy eventually reduced the hospital death rate by two-thirds. The story of Cap and Nightingale became part of the Nightingale heroic narrative. Was Cap a mystical symbol of what the founder of modern nursing was to do? Cap's story and its significance to the Florence Nightingale legend tantalize us with possibilities.

Buddy, a female German shepherd, and Morris Frank, a young man who had lost his sight, showed America that those who lacked sight did not need to be helpless. Buddy was the first Seeing Eye dog in the United States, and she and Morris Frank helped thousands of blind people achieve independence. Together Buddy and Frank helped establish a guide dog school for the blind in America and set a standard for the world to follow.

Labrador retrievers Boe and Budge pioneered the role of combat operational stress control dogs. Stigma prevents many who need help from getting mental health care. With a dog present, a therapist seemed more approachable, and the dogs assisted with the flow of therapeutic communication. The COSC dogs benefited soldiers in several ways, including destigmatizing mental health intervention.

Pioneering Therapy dogs today join health professionals in the modern health care setting. These canine workers are unique in a hospital environment in their ability to touch people, physically and psychologically. Therapy animals can provide the touch and comfort that many hospital patients need.

Terms

A variety of terms are used to describe dogs working in health care, so it is helpful, at the onset, to define the terms that this book uses to describe the roles of therapy and service dogs. The need for common terminology in animal-assisted interventions is a recurring theme in the development of animal-assisted interventions and is discussed again in Chapter 8. A list of these terms and their definitions is also provided in the glossary.

Therapy Dogs

Therapy dogs visit with a handler to provide affection and comfort to various members of the public, typically in a variety of facility settings such as hospitals, retirement homes, and schools. A therapy dog has no special rights of access, except in those facilities where they are welcomed. Therapy dog teams pass a test by a national organization that shows that the handler and animal are suitable. Therapy dog teams are volunteers, and the dogs are personal pets. They participate as part of a treatment program in animal-assisted therapy, or in less formal, social activity as animal-assisted activity.[5]

Assistance Dogs (also called Service Dogs)

"Assistance animal" is a broad term used to describe an animal supporting someone with a disability. Assistance animals are also commonly called "service animals." In this book, the term assistance dog includes all types of assistance dogs, including service dogs. An assistant or service dog has been individually trained to do work or perform tasks for an individual with a disability. The functions performed by the dog must be directly related to the person's disability. Examples include guide dogs for people who are blind, hearing dogs for people who are deaf, and dogs who provide mobility assistance or communicate medical alerts. Therapy dogs and assistance dogs (including service dogs) have different rights of access. Assistance dogs are considered working animals, not pets. Guide, hearing, and service dogs are permitted, in accordance with the Americans with Disabilities Act, to accompany a person with a disability almost anywhere the general public is allowed.[6] A guide dog is a service dog who has been trained to assist a blind or visually impaired person.

Facility Dog

A facility animal is an animal who is regularly present in a residential or clinical setting. These animals may be a variety of species, from dogs and cats to birds and fish. They might live with a handler who is an employee of the facility and come to work each day, or they might live at the facility full time under the care of a primary staff person. Facility animals should be specially trained for extended interactions with clients or residents of the facility.[7]

Chapter 8 discusses the distinctions in roles and privileges of therapy dogs, service dogs, and assistance dogs. These differences are important, but roles are often confused. Additional definitions of roles are in the glossary.

In this book, *health care* is defined as activities and efforts to promote physical and mental health and/or to maintain or restore physical or mental health, especially by licensed professionals. Health care includes activities and efforts to promote, maintain, and restore public health and community health, rehabilitation, and access to care.

The Mercy Dogs in Chapter 1 were called by many names including Red Cross Dogs. In this chapter, the term Mercy Dog will be used as a generic term. The term Red Cross Dog will be used when the reference is to a Mercy Dog working in the Red Cross.

The stories of the Dog Pioneers raise our curiosity. They reveal how a dog stepped in at one moment in history to transform health care by showing humans the power of the human-animal bond. For each of these dogs, their contribution was possible because a human was listening, watching, and learning. It was a triumph of partnership, of interspecies collaboration. The stories of the Dog Pioneers are both transformative and cautionary. The changes inspired by the Dog Pioneers are evidence of the strong bond between human and dog. As we have worked with them, we have learned about ourselves. The strong bond between human and dog creates the dog's ultimate willingness and dedication to serving us in roles from war dog to Mercy Dog to modern therapy dog.

Our relationships with them have often cost dogs a great deal. Their service and contributions prompt us to examine the different humane values and questions that emerge when humans rely on the devotion of dogs to accomplish our work and caution us with issues for the future of our inter-species collaboration. What are our responsibilities to our animal companions who so faithfully do our work out of devotion?

As humans explore the roles and stress of our dogs' experience in their work comforting and healing us, we are challenged to examine the ambiguity of our relationships with them. We view our dogs as darling objects of affec-tion and love, in need of our protection, almost like children. However, we have also used them as tools of war or service to be used for the benefit of humans regardless of the physical or emotional cost to the animal. Today the role of dogs and all animals in animal-assisted programs is evolving into a more mutually beneficial partnership. Animals are not merely "used" but instead intentionally integrated into the care system, no longer viewed as objects, but as living, breathing, and feeling members of a team.

As humans continue the arc of discovery to understand the common links we have shared with our dogs as unique interconnected creatures that share a common earth perhaps even higher gains will be achieved. The Dog Pioneers were a diverse lot but shared common traits that made each a pio-neer. What were these traits, and how did the partnership between them and a human mentor expand into a contribution in a system as complicated as human health care?

As we travel the journeys of the Dog Pioneers of health care, what might we still learn from dogs about the intersection of the human-animal bond and our shared well-being?

1

The Mercy Dogs
of World War I

The dog heard and smelled the war. The collie had first detected gunfire when he was still miles away in the base camp. The smell of smoke and gas was thousands of times stronger to the dog than to his human comrades. Now the deafening sounds and scents of gunfire engulfed him. Still, the collie crawled steadily, not stopping or resting. The dog crept on to his destination. He did not bark. He knew he must not alert the enemy.

The trench was dark and wet, and the young soldier smelled the blood pumping from his lower leg wound. He saw his best friend, Billy, still right there next to him, but now Billy lay face down in the muddy trench, shot in the head just as he had taken a last bite of breakfast. Battlefield rats as big as cats had polished off the rest of Billy's uneaten biscuit.

Now the soldier thought he saw something through the smoke. It looked like a small red cross, moving, almost floating, through the dense fog. The man's head wound throbbed. He blinked blood out of his eyes.

He saw the dog now, a small collie with a red cross on his back. The dog looked straight at him and crouched, inch-by-inch, closer and deeper into the trench to reach him. The collie wore a tattered brown satchel strapped on his back and traveled in the so-called "no man's land" between two trenches. One trench belonged to the Allies. Another trench belonging to the enemy ran parallel to the one he, Billy, and the advancing dog now shared. The soldier could see that the dog's low size helped him avoid enemy fire; the collie traveled low in a way a larger animal could not.

When the dog reached the soldier, the collie sat squarely in front of him in the trench. The soldier saw the small dog's body tremble with each crescendo of enemy fire. The dog's fur was caked with mud. The soldier reached in to release the supply bag the dog carried. The soldier leaned hard on the dog when he reached into the bag to remove the bandages. The sturdy canine shifted his weight to support the wounded man while the soldier steadied himself. The injured man applied a tourniquet and bandaged his leg wound as the dog remained still, quietly watching the human wince with each awkward effort. The dog made no sound at all except for soft panting, which the soldier could hear in the few quiet seconds in between the volleys of gunfire over their heads. Ash almost entirely covered the dog's eyes, but still the collie wagged his tail from side to side when the soldier managed to whisper "hello, boy."

The soldier's pain took over. Even in his fading consciousness, the soldier wished he had some water to give to the panting dog. He thought of his own dog, safe but so far away back home. As he closed his eyes, the soldier rested his hand on the dog's front paw. The dog stood as if at attention for a full minute, then sniffed the air a few times, turned around and crawled back through the trench the way he had come. The dog moved low and faster now.

As he closed his eyes, the soldier thought, "I am on my way home." He knew a Red Cross dog could save your life in a trench.

Canine First Responders

A dog was often the first to find a wounded soldier in World War I. The Red Cross Dogs or so-called Mercy Dogs saved thousands of soldiers' lives. In Germany, they were known as *Sanitäshunde* or Sanitary Dogs. The Allies called them by several names: Medical Dogs, Red Cross Dogs, Ambulance Dogs, and Mercy Dogs. Dogs' sense of smell and excellent night vision helped them find wounded and dying soldiers. It has been estimated that over 10,000 Red Cross or Ambulance Dogs were used on both sides in World War I. The highest numbers were used by the French and German armies.[1]

The Mercy Dogs functioned as a type of early first responder and worked as part of an ambulance unit. The dogs were marked with the Red Cross, a universally recognized medical symbol. They worked in the space between opposing forces' trenches to find and bring back wounded soldiers, an effort vital to maintaining a fighting force for the war effort. The canine recruits were trained to find injured soldiers and get as close as possible to them. Hospital corps workers might be able to see the most severely wounded men since these soldiers fell where they fought, but human rescuers might miss soldiers that still had the strength to crawl away or hunt for water or shelter. A trained Mercy Dog could work low and silently to search for men in the trenches and was trained not to bark to alert the enemy. The dogs deployed at night since the lights would expose the wounded to the enemy.

In his 1917 historical sketch of working dogs in the great war, *Scout, Red Cross and Army Dogs*, Theo. F. Jager described the roles, training, and use of dogs in World War I in a training guide for the rank and file of the United

States Army.[2] Jaeger wrote that the dogs were trained to help only those who were still alive. The objective was to sort the wounded into categories of those who could be saved and those who could not. A Mercy Dog learned to distinguish between the uniform of the enemy and his soldiers, find his wounded man, and bring news of his injured comrade back to his soldier partner. The dogs were to carry a piece of clothing of the wounded soldier back to the base location, and then they could lead the way back to the injured soldier. Each dog carried a first aid pack; when he found a wounded man, the soldier could take the package. The soldier could then help himself and would be able to tend to his wounds. Then the Mercy Dog role was to bring a message to the dog's soldier partner.[3]

If the dog did not discover a wounded man, the dog was to trot to his handler and lie down. If he had found a wounded soldier, he was trained to urge his handler to follow him to the wounded man. The German dogs had a short strap buckled to their collar and were taught to grasp the belts in their mouth and return to their unit when they found a wounded man.

Their soldier's life and the dog's life depended on the dogs' skills. However, even a mortally wounded World War I soldier need not die alone and without comfort. A faithful Mercy Dog often stayed by the dying hero's side, remaining as a last comforting comrade on the battlefield until the soldier died.

World War I was a trench war. Huge guns blew away the earth to create gaping trenches. Choking mustard gas filled the air. The trenches themselves were a thick morass of mud and blood infested with rats and insects. It was a nightmare for the men. It was a horrible place for a dog. The smells and sounds of war were intense to the canine senses. The sense of smell and acute sense of hearing create much of a dog's sense of the world. Dogs' keen auditory ability allows them to hear sounds from miles away.[4] A dog has 220 million olfactory receptors compared to 5 million in the human nose.

Mercy Dogs were often shot and killed or injured in battle. With their signature red cross, the Mercy Dogs were often easy targets for the enemy. Theo Jager reported that the enemy did not respect the Red Cross insignia for men or dogs.[5] Some Red Cross Dogs were fitted with their own gas masks.

The Mercy Dogs were part of a long line of heroic dogs in wartime that gave their all to serve humans in warfare. Ancient Greek and Roman wall writings feature attack dogs. Napoleon used dogs as guardians. Native Americans used them for centuries as pack animals, and most armies in modern times have used dogs in some way.

World War I was the first organized use of military dogs. Canines served as messenger dogs, guard dogs, scouts, ratters, and Red Cross Dogs. Small dogs served as cigarette dogs to bring cartons of cigarettes to soldiers in the field. The French, British, and Belgians by 1918 had at least 20,000 dogs on the battlefield, the Germans 30,000. The United States was the only country to take part in World War I that did not use dogs in the war effort. The American army had no organized training of military dogs when it entered the war. America's war department believed the war would soon be over and the dogs were not needed.[6] The U.S. depended on the dogs of the Allied forces. American dogs served in the Red Cross, and Americans were eager to donate their companion dogs to work in the Red Cross program. The American Red Cross began using therapy dogs following World War II with recovering soldiers and still uses therapy dogs today.

Training for the Trenches

> A Dog can travel by day or night very rapidly over ground where a man cannot go at all or can go only very slowly; and because he travels faster, and is a smaller target, a dog has a much better chance of getting through a barrage than a man. —Lt. Col. Edwin Hautenville Richardson[7]

As World War I began, Edwin Hautenville Richardson, a British army officer and leading authority on dogs, had started to realize the value of a trained dog on the battlefield. Richardson would play a pivotal role in the development and training of the working military dog.

When the war began, there were practically no military dogs attached to the British army.[8] A dog lover, Richardson saw the potential for trained dogs to help the war effort. He understood that armies of other countries were effectively using dogs for military purposes and was an advocate for England to develop a war dog program. He believed Germany utilized the most organized system of military and police dogs.[9]

He began experimenting with military police dogs in 1898 and in 1910 attempted to convince the British government to establish an official military dog program. Richardson noted that the inability of people to recognize that a dog is capable of real work and is worth taking seriously was the main stumbling block to the adequate recognition of his highly trained dogs.[10] In the early days of the war, he offered dogs for use by the military. The British army rejected his offer. He then turned to train messenger dogs to trace the wounded on the battlefield as part of ambulance units.

While he was unsuccessful in his initial attempts to train dogs for the British army, others were more interested, and Richardson offered his trained ambulance dogs to the British Red Cross Society,[11] and the Allied armies who used Richardson's dogs as ambulance dogs.

Richardson continued to pursue his vision to establish a British War Dog School. Military men who had already begun using Richardson-trained dogs in the field eventually supported him. He started to receive requests from British officers for dogs for sentry and police work, and he began to train dogs to carry messages.[12]

Colonel Richardson claimed that a well-trained dog across the trenches was faster and more effective than a human runner. Runners could sometimes take 2 or 3 hours to make a journey back from the trenches when they had to cross open country exposed to snipers, machine gun fire, or a massive barrage. Sometimes none succeeded in getting through. A dog could travel in half an hour or less. Richardson had gained an understanding of how foreign armies used dogs. He also had a unique understanding of the animals and believed that dogs were sentient, feeling beings able to reason and act with a set of basic morals. Richardson's approach was to place the psychology and this sense of morality of the animal at the center of his training method.[13] Richardson's training philosophies would eventually gain a stronger foothold in the dog world, although skepticism persisted.[14]

Richardson's war dogs had successfully proved their value as Red Cross Dogs, messengers, sentries, and patrol dogs. The English government eventually recognized the value of the Red Cross Dogs and established the British War Dog School. Richardson became the commandant of the British War Dog School and trained over 200 dogs.

Messenger dogs and Mercy Dogs trained under battlefield conditions. They needed to become accustomed to the sights and sounds of war. A training session for a Mercy Dog needed to recreate what the dog would face on the battlefield. A dog in training learned to navigate an obstacle race with a barbed wire fence, hurdles, and tree branches. A trainer would take a group of dogs up a road and then release them to race a mile home. Larger dogs might leap over obstacles in the challenge, and smaller ones might wiggle under to achieve their objective. Clever dogs might negotiate the trip through a combination of both. All approaches were acceptable if the dog reached his goal. Next, the dogs might have to pass through a thick cloud of smoke or run from burning straw. The trainees were expected to dash through these quickly, and most learned to do so barking and tail wagging. Some rookie canines had difficulty with assigned tasks. They would never be punished but were caught by handlers and expected to try again until they were successful. Training methods used positive reinforcement, not punishment. The training environment reproduced battlefield scenarios. The dogs practiced carrying supplies and wearing gas masks. The most challenging task for the canines was to run toward some soldiers lying on the ground who fired off blank cartridges at the dogs at point blank range. The dogs learned to "freeze" on the ground if hostile fire raged above and to recognize a vocabulary of sign language. War dogs learned vital commands—*Heel, Down, Retrieve. Ssss,* a whisper, was to get the dogs' attention. *Advance* sent the dog forward. *Report* taught the dog to deliver a message from an advance post. *Report-Advance* was used after the dog had been sent from the unit to bring back help. The *Guard* command was given to tell the dog to guard prisoners. The *Report-Advance* command was the most important for the Red Cross Dogs.[15]

Each dog carried a first aid pack. When a dog discovered a wounded man, the dog was trained to allow the soldier to take the package. The soldier could then help himself and would be able to tend to his wounds. The role of the Mercy Dog was to find, stabilize, bring a message to the handler, and lead help back to the injured soldier.

The dogs were also taught to carry something from the wounded soldier back to the base location, and then they could lead the way back to the injured soldier. They were to retrieve a cap, glove, some piece of clothing from a wounded man, or a piece of grass or stone from his surroundings. This would indicate to the dog's partner back at base camp that a wounded soldier was found and awaiting aid. Although the dogs were good soldiers, they didn't always get it right. Seeking the first thing available, some dogs retrieved a temporary dressing the soldier had just used to bind his wound. The training methods were then revised to clarify orders for the obedient canine soldiers.

Search, Rescue, Triage

Involvement in the war had dramatic consequences for the mental and physical health of the men and the dogs. When World War I began and men fought in trenches, there was no organized system to identify and evacuate wounded who had a chance to survive if they could get to medical care. Men and dogs were about to partner to save lives on the battlefield.

As the role of the medical war dog was evolving, so was the new concept of battlefield medical triage. Mercy Dogs had learned to differentiate between the slightly wounded man and a soldier who was beyond help or near death. Their mission was to alert the troops back at the ambulance base camp that a man who had a chance to be saved was lying on the battlefield awaiting help.

Triage is the screening and classification of casualties to maximize the survival and welfare of patients and to make the best use of treatment resources. The word *triage* stems from the French word meaning to select or sort. Triage is a system of prioritizing treatment based on the severity of injuries, in which first responders sort out and prioritize the wounded.[16] It is a method of sorting patients by their need for treatment versus their likelihood of surviving. Modern triage is used today to determine the sequence of treatment in emergency rooms, in disasters, and on the battlefield.

The ability to triage the wounded was a crucial skill in a trench war. The survival of a soldier depended on the prompt medical treatment of battlefield wounds. Soldiers who were injured but capable of fighting again needed to be dispatched to medical care, treated, and returned to the front as quickly as possible. The survival of less severely wounded soldiers was crucial. Rapid evacuation of the wounded to early treatment became a priority. This created great challenges. Just getting away from the battle was the first step and might take days if an injured man tried to crawl to safety without help or transport. The more seriously wounded must be removed on a stretcher, but the less serious could be led out by the rescuers, some of whom had been alerted by a dog that an injured man was waiting for help back in the line of fire. Even with help, it could take hours to find the wounded and still more to transport them to adequate medical care. The path out of danger was treacherous and time was of the essence. Shell fragments lodged in wounds or tore through organs and bone. Powerful guns ripped through body parts. Mustard-colored poison gas poured into the trenches. Medical teams had to find injured men, transport them to a safe area, assess them, and treat their injuries with minimal resources. In treating trauma, a delay might mean the difference between life and death from hemorrhage, brain injury, and exposure to infection. Time meant life.

At the beginning of the war, Antoine Depage, a Belgian Royal Surgeon, introduced a defined orderly system of triage or sorting of wounded which set guidelines for evacuation and wound management. The five-step protocol, the *Ordre de Triage*, was introduced to and used by the French and Belgian armies. Robert Danis, a Depage colleague, aided in the management of the ambulance corps to transport the wounded. Together Danis and Depage established processes that provided foundations and principles of triage management. Battlefield medical evacuation consisted of a graduated system of increasingly sophisticated medical treatment posts, each further away from the battlefront. The first stop would be a Regimental Aid Post, followed by a mobile Advanced Dressing Station, where injuries could be dressed, basic care provided, or in extreme cases limb amputations performed. Medical officers had to prioritize whom to treat first.[17]

Casualties were divided into three groups. Slightly hurt soldiers could be sent back to fight. Those needing greater care were taken to field hospitals on the front line. The last to be seen were those determined to be too injured to save. In the first order of triage, the stretcher-bearers evacuated the wounded under cover of darkness. Both stretcher-bearers and their patients were exposed to gun and mortar fire. The second order of triage occurred at the clearing station, where dressings were applied, and a priority of evacuation was established before transport. Major or minor surgery was avoided at this point. For significant bleeding or wounds of the thorax, the soldier was placed in a wheelbarrow and wheeled to the safest area where an ambulance could reach him for transport. The third, fourth, and fifth orders of triage dispatched the wounded via increasingly mobile methods of treatment and evacuation.

For some wounded, the search and retrieval by the dogs began the triage process. The Mercy Dogs led the way to shorten the time from injury to treatment and created an opportunity to treat wounded men who might have been left to die of their wounds. A World War I surgeon told of the dogs' unique contribution:

> They sometimes lead us to the bodies we think have no life in them, but when we bring them back to the doctors ... they always find a spark. It is purely a matter of their instinct, [which] is far more effective than man's reasoning powers.[18]

There were other, less visible, war injuries. By the winter of 1914–15, "shell shock" had become a pressing medical and military problem in the war.[19] This signature injury of the war was a syndrome of human combat stress reaction. The term "shell shock" was coined by the soldiers themselves. Some believed it was a direct effect of exploding shells. Symptoms included fatigue, tremor, confusion, nightmares, and impaired sight and hearing. It was often diagnosed when a soldier was unable to function, and no apparent cause could be identified. Combat stress reaction was commonly viewed as a lack of moral fiber.[20] Many military officials were convinced the soldiers were malingering or cowards. Shellshocked soldiers were not able to fight, but soldiers needed to return to the front as soon as possible. Psychiatrists attempted to preserve fighting power while reducing the impact of disabling psychiatric symptoms with limited success. Some leading British psychiatrists believed the condition was psychological in nature and developed psychological interventions for treatment.[21]

Today, we appreciate the intense physical and behavioral stress of war that soldiers may experience. The Mercy Dogs also endured these stressors. Like their human comrades, the Mercy Dogs may have suffered what we describe as traumatic stress. Postwar care of the Mercy Dogs did not include concepts of stress reduction or help with trauma recovery. Dogs were viewed as loyal and eager to do their part in the service of their human "master" by their very nature.

Mercy Dogs as Patriots

> *I already have three sons and a son-in-law with the colors; now I give up my dog, and "Vive la France!"*—Communication of a father on record with the French War Office[22]

Mercy Dogs and Red Cross Dogs became a symbol of patriotism.[23] The Red Cross Dogs and other war dogs were portrayed in sentimental ways in the media; they were elevated to heroic levels and attributed human emotions and characteristics.

In a 1921 article in *Harper's* magazine, Ernest Baynes called the dogs that served in World War I "most anxious to serve."[24] In *The Red Cross Magazine* in 1917,[25] Ellwood Hendrick told of the valor and courage of Red Cross Dog Prusco, a French dog credited with saving the lives of more than 100 men who would have been left to die on the battlefield. Prusco found men who were too weak to make their location known or who were concealed by brush. Three Frenchmen were said to have been saved by Prusco when he dragged them to shelter by letting them grab his collar and pulling each one to safety. Prusco waited while each took first aid supplies from his pack and then returned to save others.

Dogs in war roles became heroes. Caesar, a bulldog who was the mascot of a company of the Fourth Battalion New Zealand Rifle Company, is memorialized in the Auckland War Memorial Museum. Caesar and his handler Rifleman Samuel Tooman traveled to Egypt in 1916 and were trained as a Red Cross ambulance team. Like all Red Cross Dogs, Caesar had to be taught to get used to the sounds of war. It was especially tricky for a bulldog to be low in the trenches because of his short, stubby body. Caesar carried medical supplies on his back, as well as writing material so the soldier could write a message and tell comrades at the base camp where the enemy was. Caesar located many wounded who might have died if they had not been rescued. Caesar reportedly was killed in action. He was found shot by a sniper, lying next to a soldier who had died with his hand resting on Caesar's head.[26] Like many Red Cross Dogs who remained with dying soldiers, Caesar and the soldier he found did not die alone. A fictionalized version of Caesar's story was later told by Patricia Stroud in her children's book, *Caesar: The Anzac Dog.*

Sergeant Stubby was a mascot war dog who received national attention, was photographed with General Pershing, and received a three-column obituary in the *New York Times.*[27] Ann Bausam's 2014 biography of Sergeant Stubby described the bond between Stubby and an American soldier and how Stubby won the heart of a nation.[28]

Legacy: Patriots in Search, Rescue, Triage

> *We have let daddy go to fight the Kaiser, and now we are sending Jack to do his bit.*—A little girl, sending her dog to the War Dog School writing to Colonel Richardson[29]

The anthropomorphic projection of human characteristics of heroism and emotion and single-mindedness of purpose onto their dogs helped humans feel better about their war effort. However, it was not so beneficial for the dogs.

Many different breeds served in the war, depending on the job at hand. Shepherds, bulldogs, farm collies, Jack Russell terriers, and Dobermans all saw action. Most dogs had a medium build and were gray or black, colors that would not be seen as well under cover of darkness. At the beginning of the war, dogs were recruited from dog shelters such as the Home for Lost Dogs at Battersea or from police forces. The breeds requested were sheepdogs, collies, Irish terriers, lurchers, Welsh terriers, and deerhounds.[30]

Later, a public call went out for dogs to "do their bit." Thousands of American dogs were donated to the war effort through the Red Cross or the war dog programs of other nations. In fact, Americans were eager to donate companion dogs to serve in the war. Thousands of American families said goodbye to their companions to send them off to an uncertain fate, feeling they were doing a patriotic and heroic thing. A November 1917 note in the *Red Cross Magazine* announced that more dogs were needed for the war effort.[31] Just two months later, in January 1918, the Red Cross issued a notice of "no more dogs needed"[32] because so many companion dogs had been donated. It is not known how many, if any, of these pets returned to their families or what life held for them after the war.

Our relationship with war dogs raises questions about the attachment of humans and dogs. What was the emotional cost to families to surrender their dogs to a war effort that was likely to cost that pet injury or death? Did they hope to see them again? Did they believe their companion animals could volunteer? Why do dogs serve us so faithfully in such hazardous conditions?

The Mercy Dogs were part of a long line of heroic dogs in wartime that gave their all to serve humans in war. When trench warfare ended, the skills of dogs that could navigate the trenches were no longer needed, but dogs remained active parts of war. It is likely that men will continue to have battles in which dogs will faithfully and heroically serve by their side.

Dogs and humans who are companions in war form an intimate relationship. The man and the dog are both ready to give their lives in the performance of their duty. But it is a partnership developed to suit a human purpose.

There may be more lessons to learn about our responsibility in our human-animal collaboration. Dogs do not volunteer to serve in a war. However, they serve us with their full measure of devotion. This raises humane questions. Do we understand how war affects our canine soldiers? What is our appropriate role in this mutual bond with dogs who serve beside us?

The American Veterinary Medical Association defines the human-animal bond as a "mutually beneficial and dynamic relationship between people and other animals, influenced by behaviors essential to the health and well-being of both."[33] As part of this reciprocal bond, fulfilling our human responsibility to provide for the safety and well-being of our working animal partners implies balancing our human needs with the dogs' needs and nature.

Since World War I, dogs have been deployed into combat, yet we have not fully understood the impact of this setting and the work we assign to our canine partners. Modern researchers are now exploring this issue. Some recent studies have shown that not being able to predict what happens next can be a significant stressor for dogs as well as humans. Dogs placed in war or battlefield settings may repeatedly be subjected to stressors. Combat-related behavioral issues developed by combat dogs were given the name canine posttraumatic stress disorder within the past decade.[34]

The Mercy Dogs of World War I taught us how to collaborate with dogs to care for our wounded in the most challenging of conditions. The Mercy Dogs inspired new search and rescue techniques as we developed new systems of triage on the battlefield. They showed us that communication and mutual comfort between dog and man do not need words, even in the most chaotic environment and even at the end of life. Why do our dogs serve us so faithfully even in such hazardous and what must be terrifying situations? Colonel

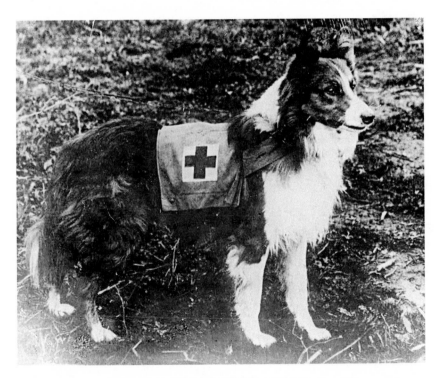

A Red Cross Dog waits to "do his bit," Italy, 1909 (Library of Congress).

Richardson wrote "that in the dog, I have found ... love to be the motive power most successful in obtaining good results."[35] Affection for us and reward are central to our bond with dogs, and it is that bond that makes them so willing to serve us. The dogs of war showed us how training and partnership between man and dog could and should benefit both.

As World War I ended, the Mercy Dogs' role drifted into history, but the winds of war would soon blow again. As a Nazi threat loomed over the world, Jofi, Sigmund Freud's chubby chow, would soon step into the father of psychoanalysis's consulting room to demonstrate another way a dog could promote healing and understanding in perilous times.

2

Jofi and Sigmund Freud

The curved stone staircase led to two doors at the top of the landing. American poet Hilda Doolittle chose the door on the right, the one that opened to Sigmund Freud's consulting room. Doolittle crossed the threshold, scanned the room, and prepared to meet the famous psychoanalyst. She was fascinated by Freud's antiquities. Precious objets d'art stood precisely arranged, sharing a semicircular space with a series of vases, each with a single flower or a spray of orchids. The office was not the sterile, sparse workspace one might expect for the pioneer of psychoanalysis. A plain divan-style couch sat with a rug folded at its foot. An old-fashioned porcelain stove stood at the foot of the couch. Doolittle heard no sound from the Vienna street outside. A window in the consulting room and one in the other room looked out on the courtyard.[1]

As the American poet waited to meet the famous doctor, another Freud treasure approached, one as legendary as the professor himself and Freud's collection of antiquities.[2] *Freud's chow dog Jofi greeted Doolittle. In her* Tribute to Freud, *the poet recalled:*

A little lion-like creation emerges from under the couch and came padding toward me. I bend down to greet the creature, but Freud says, "do not touch her— she snaps—she is very difficult with strangers."[3]

Doolittle did not consider herself a dog lover but knew that dogs sometimes liked her and decided to take the risk. Continuing her gesture toward the little chow, Doolittle crouched on the floor so that Jofi could snap better if she wanted to. Doolittle recalled,

"Jofi snuggles her nose into my hand and nuzzles her head against my shoulder."[4]

Jofi granted Doolittle immediate acceptance, and the poet began her analysis. Jofi continued to play a central role in Hilda Doolittle's analysis.[5]

For four days a week from 5:00 to 6:00 in the afternoon, and one day a week from noon to 1:00,[6] *Sigmund Freud psychoanalyzed Doolittle as she reclined on the famous couch in his study. Outside the window, on the streets of Vienna, clouds of the Holocaust gathered. Doolittle wrote, "Occasional coquettish, confetti-like showers from the air, gilded paper swastikas floated through the streets."[7]*

As the skies darkened over Vienna, the 77-year-old Jewish psychoanalyst sat out of sight behind the famous couch, smoked a cigar, and excavated the archeology of the 6-foot-tall, 47-year-old American poet's unconscious. Underneath the couch sat a lion-like chubby chow with a hearty appetite and an impeccable sense of timing.

Each, in their way, changed history.

Sigmund Freud: Dog Lover

Sigmund Freud appreciated the comforting presence of dogs in his life. He and his family shared their life with many dogs, including a Chow-Chow named Jofi (pronounced Yofi). Freud played with his family dogs and received birthday cards from them every year written in poetry by his daughter Anna.[8] During Freud's illness, he had difficulty chewing because of jaw cancer, and Jofi often finished his plate.[9] Freud was also beginning to understand his dog's potential for therapeutic inquiry in the consulting room.

Sigmund Freud was an Austrian neurologist and a prolific writer, scholar, and thinker. He developed the foundations of psychoanalytical theory and is generally considered the father of modern-day psychoanalysis. Freud's theories influenced generations of psychotherapists. Although the theory and practice of modern psychoanalysis evolved, Freud provided the foundations that remain today.[10]

Sigmund Freud was born in 1856 in the Austrian town of Freiberg. Freud's family moved to Vienna when he was 4 years old, and he lived and worked there most of his life. Freud married Martha Bernays, and together they had six children. Anna, his youngest, was analyzed by Freud and became a psychoanalyst. Freud published volumes of writings, including thousands of letters.

To develop his work, Freud collaborated with others, including Josef Breuer, Carl Jung, Alfred Adler, Karl Abraham, and Otto Rank. However, at the onset of the Second World War, Freud was increasingly disillusioned. He had philosophical differences and rivalries with several of his colleagues. The political world was growing ominous. In 1933, the Nazis burned some of Freud's books, causing him to remark, "What progress we are making. In the Middle Ages, they would have burned me. And now they are content with burning my books."[11]

At the time of the poet Hilda Doolittle's analysis, Freud was old, frail, and ill, but he was still working, seeing patients and writing.[12] Freud seemed to be a man of contradictions. On the one hand, he was a bitter, pessimistic old man with a sharp wit, often cruel to critics; on the other hand, he had a capacity for great kindness and tenderness. It was his interactions with Jofi and his other dogs that perhaps best revealed the father of psychoanalysis's more tender side, especially towards the end of his life. In 1938, Freud and his wife and daughter fled Vienna for England to escape the Nazis. He had developed throat cancer but never quit smoking. He was said to have smoked over 20 cigars a day, and his daily walks included a trip to the cigar store. He underwent more than 30 operations and eventually died in 1939.

Psychoanalytical Theory

To understand Jofi's pioneering role as Freud's canine assistant, an understanding of the fundamental principles and practices of Freudian psychoanalysis is helpful. What was this new art and science of Freud's psychoanalysis, and how could a dog play a role?

Psychoanalysis examines what is beneath the surface of human behavior. In Freudian psychoanalysis, the analyst's role is to use the dynamics of the therapeutic relationship to facilitate patient insight into and to encourage free expression of feelings, especially repressed feelings. Psychoanalysis developed from an understanding of Freud and his contemporaries of the power of talking about questions and issues that are difficult to understand. Freud was curious about what motivates people and causes them to act in ways that are counter to their own interest.

The relationship between the patient and the analyst is at the heart of analytical therapy and allows the examination of unconscious factors by examining the therapy relationship in the present experience. The goals of analysis are to help the patient access the unconscious and let go of repressed feelings and emotions. Freud's theories on the development of the unconscious and conscious mind, the structure of personality, stages of psychosexual development, defense mechanisms, and dream interpretation were vital contributions to psychology.

The psychoanalytic theory holds that people are to a great degree unaware of why they feel or act in a certain way.[13] Freud's theories recognize the influence of the unconscious, dreams, and emotional trauma in the development of mental symptoms. Freud believed he could help a patient uncover repressed or hidden conflicts related to past events through a process called free association with a trained analyst to interpret and encourage the expression of the content. Psychoanalysis is an intense process. The analysis in Freud's era and still today usually involves several weekly visits.

Mark Edmundson has described the fundamental perception of Freud's work. "At the center of Freud's work was a fundamental perception: human beings are not unified beings. Our psyches are not whole but divided into parts, and those parts are usually in conflict with each other."[14]

Freud theorized that the mind was divided into the id, the ego, and the superego. The unconscious id is the part of the mind that stores thoughts, feelings, and urges; although the conscious individual is unaware of these things, the content influences his or her experiences. The ego functions as a sort of go-between for the id, the center of primitive impulses for self-preservation, and the superego or conscience. The superego is the component of personality needed to function in the world and in areas such as perception, evaluation, and judgment. The ego must negotiate a frequently hostile outside world.[15] Defense mechanisms—which include denial, repression, and projection—are used by the ego to deal with conflict. Dreams, another part of the Freudian theory, allow individuals to respond to unconscious demands while sleeping. Through imagery and hallucinations, dreams provide a window into the unconscious.

The concepts of repression, resistance, and free association are fundamental to an understanding of the psychoanalytical practice and how Freud integrated Jofi into his analytical work. Freud used his observations of his patient's reactions to Jofi to encourage expression of repressed psychological issues. Repression is a defense where an individual's impulses and instinctual desires are blocked from consciousness. It is a process of unconsciously blocking ideas or memories that are viewed as unacceptable. Resistance is a patient's unconscious opposition to exploring painful memories or content during psychoanalysis. Free association is the process whereby the patient tells the story of his or her life by just saying whatever comes to mind.[16]

Psychoanalytical treatment is based on the principle that people are motivated by unconscious wishes and desires. These can be brought into conscious awareness by examining the real-time, present relationship between patient and analyst. By observing the patient's interaction with others and listening to the patient feely share dreams and fantasies, the analyst has a unique perspective on the patient. The analyst listens for patterns and themes, which provide clues to the repressed content and sources of resistance.

The analyst's couch often symbolized the process of psychoanalysis, with its focus on uncovering and confronting unconscious content.[17] A couch was used based on the premise that a patient would be more relaxed if he or she were resting comfortably, out of sight of the analyst. Not being able to see the analyst was thought to stimulate free association so that the analyst was a blank screen upon which the patient's thoughts, fantasies, dreams, and other conscious and unconscious content could be projected, uncontaminated by reality.

As part of the psychoanalytic process, the patient develops a relationship with the analyst called transference, which also is analyzed. Analyzing the transference and countertransference helps to uncover unconscious factors that drive present behavior. Transference and countertransference are tools in psychoanalytical work. Transference is the projection onto another person (the analyst) of feelings, past associations, and experiences. It is important because it demonstrates that experiences influence the present, and interpreting transference in the psychoanalytic setting can shed light on unresolved conflicts.[18] Countertransference is the analyst's or therapist's feelings and attitudes towards the patient and his or her reaction to the patient's transference. The analyst can see how his or her own experience influences the understanding of the patient and recognize his or her emotional responses to the patient.[19]

Freud's work has been both widely criticized and praised but has profoundly impacted psychological theory development and practice. Many contemporaries of Freud felt that he put too much emphasis on sexuality and that his approach was scandalous. This criticism provoked a feeling of disloyalty and abandonment in Freud, who valued loyalty.

Understanding these principles of psychoanalytical theory, we might well wonder: What part could a charismatic chow play in this new and intense psychoanalysis?

Jofi: Shock Absorber Who Snores

Jofi was a constant presence in Freud's consulting room and became part of the psychoanalytical process. Freud observed the patient's reaction to Jofi and used his interpretation of these reactions to encourage the patient's expression of unconscious content. Freud's chow became a conduit for communication, a symbol, and comfort to the ill and aging Freud. As Freud's patients explored the storms on the horizon of their unconscious, their reactions to a free-roaming lion-like chow under the couch became a sort of furry barometer of the analytical weather.

Freud and Jofi thus became true pioneers in interspecies learning and collaboration. Freud explored new ways to access unconscious content, new therapeutic tools, and new approaches. As Freud watched Jofi, he theorized about dogs' ability to sense and evoke emotions. Freud's ability and willingness to integrate his dog into his therapeutic process may have been due to a combination of Freud's affection for dogs, his view of them as sentient beings, his trust in their reactions, and his openness to experiencing them as species who could teach humans about their own human nature.

Freud said he thought dogs were superior to people because they did not struggle with ambiguity. He admired dogs' loyalty. Ambivalence was a fundamental concept for Freud. For Freud, all intimate relationships were ambivalent and involved both love and hate. His daughter Anna Freud quoted her father as professing, "Dogs love their friends and bite their enemies, quite unlike people who are incapable of pure love and always have to mix love and hate."[20] Freud thought that dogs' nature was pure.[21]

Many a dog lover might admit to singing an occasional tune to their canine companion and the father of psychoanalysis was no exception. Freud sang to Jofi. Freud admitted much sentiment and comfort attached to his relationship to Jofi: "Often when stroking Jofi, I have caught myself humming a melody which unmusical as I am, I can't help recognizing the aria from Don Giovanni. A bond of friendship unites us both."[22]

Like so many dogs who seem to find their human guardians just when the human is ready to learn the lessons the dog can teach, Jofi seemed to enter Freud's life when he may have most needed her. Freud's love of dogs came to him later in life. In the mid–1920s, as Freud approached 70 years old, Wolf, the dog of his daughter Anna, joined the family and Freud was smitten. A friend of Anna Freud gave Freud a chow named Lün-Yu in 1928. Unfortunately, Lün-Yu died after 15 months. Jofi was Lün-Yu's sister, and when she joined Freud, she becomes his treasured companion.[23]

Today we might be tempted to call the father of psychoanalysis an unabashed "pet parent." Dogs were an essential part of family life in the Freud home. Anna began a tradition of writing poems to her father in the persona of the dog. On Freud's birthday, Anna would attach a sign that said "happy birthday" to a dog's collar and send the dog in to greet her father. When Jofi became pregnant, Freud remarked that one of the litter would be given away, but one would be kept by him and "become a Freud," indicating he viewed Jofi's offspring as a member of the family and perhaps a modern-day grand-dog. In the end, one of Jofi's puppies survived, and Freud kept him. Dogs revealed Freud's tender side.

Many of Freud's patients remarked that the combination of dog smell and cigar smoke made the experience in Freud's consulting room memorable.[24] Meeting Jofi for the first time was likely to be a defining moment for any new Freud patient. The face that no doubt greeted visitors as they arrived and began their free association was that of a scowling lion-like Chow with the charisma of a teddy bear.

Chows are highly intelligent and dignified and value their independence. They also have a frowning expression, which may appear like a scowl. The chow is one of the oldest breeds[25] thought to come from China, and it is often recognizable in Chinese pottery and sculpture. In fact, Hilda Doolittle remarked on the resemblance of a Coptic clay artifact to Jofi when Freud showed it to her.[26] The statue was even the same color as Jofi.

For patients of the great doctor, Jofi may well have seemed as formidable as the professor himself did as she moved freely around Freud's office and home with her beautiful high-set tail and distinctive stiff gait. A Chow moves her back legs like stilts and moves rapidly. The almond eyes of a Chow can give a mysterious look, quiet and thoughtful, perhaps resembling the great professor himself. A mid-sized dog, chows usually weigh from 45 to 70 pounds; with their relatively equal length and height (each about 18 inches), their body has a square appearance.[27]

In his consulting room, the father of psychoanalysis could not ignore the chubby chow. Neither could his patients, as the following excerpt from Hilda Doolittle's letter to Conrad Aiken confirms.

> His room was filled with orchids. He has a passion for chows. Has Yo-fi always in the room. Fortunately, Yofi took to me; otherwise, I should have fled in anguish. She was pregnant, sat on the chair and helped with the analysis—sort of a shock absorber.[28]

Hilda Doolittle

Hilda Doolittle was a 20th-century American poet who was analyzed by Sigmund Freud from 1933 to 1934. Doolittle wrote under her initials "H. D." She is well known for her poetry but also wrote memoirs, short stories, essays, reviews, and a children's book. She was the first woman to receive the Award of Merit Medal for Poetry from the American Academy of Arts and Letters in 1960.

In 1911 Doolittle emigrated to England, and in 1913 she married Richard Aldington. She and Aldington later separated but remained friends throughout their lives. In 1916, H. D. met Bryher (Annie Winifred Ellerman), a wealthy English novelist and the daughter of a wealthy shipping magnate; Bryher then became the most significant enduring relationship in Doolittle's life. Bryher and H. D. lived together and were companions, although they both had other partners. Doolittle's first child had been born stillborn, her brother was killed in the war, and she was estranged from her husband when she approached Freud in Vienna. She sought analysis due to anxiety about the rise of Hitler and the series of personal losses and tragedies she had experienced, as well as a block in her writing. Freud's analysis of Doolittle occurred when he was in his 70s, toward the end of his career. The poet was in her 40s and at the peak of her career.

During this period, Doolittle wrote of her analysis in letters to friends, sometimes several letters a day. Many letters were to Bryher.[29] The analysis was a crucial event in Doolittle's life, and she mentioned it repeatedly in her letters.[30] These letters provide one of the most detailed descriptions of what occurred in the analysis. She also wrote of her experience of psychoanalysis in her book, *Tribute to Freud*.[31]

Adam Phillips, writing in the introduction to *Tribute to Freud*, described

Doolittle's book as "a piece of writing so artfully akin to a patient speaking from the couch"; he added that psychoanalysts today might be surprised by how "unorthodox a Freudian Freud was."[32] As reflected in Doolittle's account, Freud's own style of analysis was surprisingly informal compared to modern standards of analytical psychiatry or the rules he established for his followers. Freud's relationship with Doolittle exceeded the boundaries of what is traditionally accepted in the therapeutic relationship, in which the analyst takes the stance of a blank screen. Freud showed Doolittle around the room, exchanged gifts with her, loaned her books, and was "tender" with her, as she described in her letters. They talked about the dog in the room.

Doolittle's letters, poems, and books provide a spotlight into her experience with the father of psychoanalysis[33] and allow us to meet Jofi, observe the remarkable chow's partnership with Freud, and see firsthand Jofi's role in the analytical process. Reports and descriptions of the various roles and antics of Jofi and other dogs in the Freud consulting room also appear in the letters of Anna Freud and Freud's colleagues, family, and patients.[34] Freud himself never wrote about using his dogs in the analysis, but his writings, diaries, and works include numerous references to his dogs in his personal life and his affection for them. From March 1930 to January 1937, references to Jofi appeared in Freud's journals, letters, and memorabilia.[35] Family snapshots and home movies included Jofi.

Several biographies of Freud and papers about his life and work mentioned the fondness he had for his dogs and their importance to him in his family life and in his analytical work.[36] Several Freud biographers said that Jofi sat quietly by Freud's couch. Biographer Peter Gay mentioned Jofi only in passing and seemed less impressed with her presence therapeutically. Gay reported that Freud and Jofi were inseparable and Jofi would sit quietly at the foot of the couch during analytical sessions. Other biographers and correspondents of Freud described a more active and free-roaming Jofi.

Writing in "Freud's Damn Dog," Showalter[37] reported a secondhand anecdote from his teacher Roy Grinker, Sr., who was analyzed by Freud from 1933 to 1935. Grinker, who founded the psychiatry program at Michael Reese Hospital in Chicago, had been a patient of Freud and recalled that Jofi and Anna's dog would start barking when anyone ran to the doorbell and that the dogs had the run of the office and the shared waiting room. Grinker reported that the Wolfhound would sniff at Grinker's genitals and that he thus entered Freud's office "with a high degree of castration anxiety."[38]

Jofi would sit beside Grinker and scratch at the door when she wanted to get out. After Freud let Jofi out, he would comment to Grinker that Jofi hadn't thought much about what Grinker had been talking about. When Jofi returned, Freud remarked that Jofi had granted Grinker a second chance. Grinker also reported that in one session where he was expressing strong emotion, the "damn dog jumped on top of me." Freud told Grinker that Jofi was excited that Grinker "had explored the roots of his anxiety."[39]

Doolittle's writing reflects some mixed feelings and a sense of competing for affection with the Chow, all of which became grist for Freud's therapeutic mill. In her *Tribute to Freud,* Doolittle observed, "I was annoyed at the end of my session as Jofi would wander about and I felt the professor was more interested in Jofi than in my story."[40] Doolittle added, "One never knows what he is about to embark on but he is most keen on dogs, and one of his chows walked out on me the last hour."[41]

Freud integrated Jofi into his sessions by reflecting on how she engaged with the patient and how the patient reacted to her when she did. For example, Freud might comment on a reaction to a patient's free association: "Jofi doesn't approve of what you are saying."[42] Freud became interested in Jofi's reaction to his patients. He noticed that Jofi would become restless if the patient was dealing with anger or anxiety. He saw that the presence of the dog in the consulting room reduced tension, especially with children or adolescents. Jofi would sit further away from the patient depending on how anxious the patient was. If the patient was depressed, Jofi sat closer.

Jofi apparently multitasked in her role in the office. She developed into a timekeeper for the father of psychiatry. The psychotherapeutic hour then, as now, is typically 50 minutes. This break allows the therapist to take notes, take a break for personal needs, and reflect on the session. Jofi would move toward the door as the 50-minute time approached, and Freud would know it was time to end the session without looking at his clock. In his memoir of his father, Martin Freud recalled that Jofi would signal the end of the therapy hour by getting up to yawn.[43]

Jofi could also be distracting to the patient. In one session, Doolittle complained that Jofi lay on the floor and snored loudly for nearly the entire session.[44] Doolittle also recalled an episode in which Jofi drank water under the table and then went to sleep and moaned and sobbed during her nap. Freud stopped Doolittle from talking and explained that Jofi was pregnant and having strange dreams.[45]

Topsy: A Symbolic Story

Dogs were often symbols and metaphors for Freud. Another dog, Topsy, would be symbolic in Freud's life. *Topsy: A Golden Haired Chow* was a book by Marie Bonaparte, a Freud analysand, friend, and benefactor. Bonaparte had introduced Freud to a love of dogs, while Freud introduced Bonaparte to psychoanalysis. During World War II, Bonaparte would ransom the Freud family out of Austria.

From 1937 to 1938, while the two were hounded by the Gestapo in Vienna, Freud and his daughter Anna collaborated to translate Bonaparte's book on Topsy into German. Freud and Anna translated the book out of gratitude to Bonaparte and because of their shared love for dogs. Being engaged in this work temporarily distracted Freud from his concern about the Nazi political situation in Vienna, as well as his own failing health. He was growing restless and increasingly perceived his colleagues as disloyal.

Topsy is a tale of the effects of a dog on its owner and reflects the psychoanalytical impact of relationships with animals. The book *Topsy* placed a spotlight on issues such as grieving, mourning, and transience. *Topsy* became a metaphor for Freud at this challenging time. It was a dog story with profound symbolism for Freud.

The book also was thought to have a historical context. Written in France and Greece at the onset of World War II, the story of Topsy's cancer was thought to convey the ills of Europe at that time. W. L. Reiser, writing in "Topsy—Living and Dying: A Footnote to History," stated that the book *Topsy* reveals relationships between Freud, Anna, and Bonaparte and Freud's struggle with his own illness.[46] Topsy was a chow who struggled with jaw cancer, and Freud also had jaw cancer; both were treated with radiation. In the story, the owner of Topsy discovers how much she has become attached to the dog only after she learns he is suffering from jaw cancer.

Jofi's Legacy: A New Kind of Partnership

Freud and Jofi were the first animal-assisted therapy partnership in psychotherapy. A psychoanalyst's role is to assist the patient to become consciously aware of unconscious patterns that impair functioning. Jofi introduced the concept that a dog could help a therapist guide a patient's journey of self-discovery and that a dog might act as a social lubricant for patients.

His beloved chow originally accompanied Freud in his consulting office to provide comfort to Freud, who claimed Jofi helped him relax in the session. Freud then noticed that the dog also helped his patients relax, especially children and adolescents. The famous psychoanalyst watched his dog, and he learned. Freud accepted Jofi for the dog that she was and observed her effect on himself and his patients.

We cannot know for certain what Jofi may have experienced in her collaboration with Freud, but we can appreciate her legacy in animal-assisted psychotherapy. Freud and Jofi ultimately provided validation of the benefit of pets in individual psychotherapy to a skeptical psychological profession. However, the journey to full acceptance of animal-assisted intervention in psychotherapy would take decades.

Stanley Coren, professor in the Department of Psychology at the University of British Columbia, wrote about Freud's work with Jofi in the foreword to Aubrey Fine's *Handbook on Animal-Assisted Therapy*.[47] Coren explained that during analysis, patients experience resistance; they might become hostile or stop sharing feelings or information. This blockage or resistance must be worked through as part of the analytical work. Freud observed that a dog in the room could decrease expressions of this resistance. Freud speculated on the reasons for this and concluded that the dog's neutral, nonjudgmental reaction to anything the patient said, even if it was something very embarrassing or painful, gave the patient confidence and a feeling of acceptance and reassurance. Freud then encouraged the systematic use of his dogs in therapy.[48]

The analysand's reaction to Jofi also provided the opportunity for Freud to comment on what he observed and explore its meaning with the patient. Patients may have experienced feelings of acceptance or rejection from Jofi, which may have found their way into their free association of feelings. Jofi may have stimulated more trust in Freud as a therapist, reducing tension and humanizing the blank screen of the famous analyst. In some cases, Jofi may have frightened or threatened the patient, especially one who was not a dog lover, and this anxiety may have also brought the patient into the here and now of the relationship with the analyst.

For Freud's patients, Jofi provided a sort of icebreaker, a communication channel, an object of transference of their inner feelings, and perhaps even a spyglass into the softer side of Freud. Hilda Doolittle best described the effect of the dog in the consulting room when she called Jofi a sort of "shock absorber."[49] Doolittle proposed that as Jofi sat in a chair at her feet, perhaps she had been trained to give the patient confidence.[50]

For Freud himself, Jofi was a symbol of affection, loyalty, and fidelity and unambiguous interspecies friendship. Freud and Jofi's partnership provided the foundation for the emergence of animal-assisted psychotherapy. Jofi's legacy was to become a symbol of the validation of the benefit of animals in therapeutic encounters. Without Jofi's story, the acceptance of animal-assisted therapy might not have occurred decades later when another psychologist, Boris Levinson, presented his own findings from working with his own dog, Jingles.

Fine, in *The Handbook of Animal-Assisted Therapy*, explained that animals can serve as a social lubricant for therapy.[51] Animal-assisted therapy is based on emotional connections and evolving therapeutic relationships present in the therapy room.[52] An animal's presence may contribute to a perception of a safe environment; patients who feel that the therapist is caring for the animal and makes the dog feel safe may trust the therapist to do the same for them. Animals can also be seen as an extension of the therapist. They provide enthusiastic greetings to most patients.[53] The mere presence of an animal in the room can evoke emotions—humorous emotions and a wide range of others. A snoring chow is difficult to ignore in a therapeutic session.

An animal may be permitted to display feelings towards the patient that may not be appropriate for an analyst to display, such as hugging, cuddling, or yawning, and in the process provide much-needed comfort or reassurance.

Jofi's work with Freud pioneered the way for future collaboration between psychotherapists and their dogs. In the 1960s, American psychologist Boris Levinson introduced and documented the way companion animals could help develop therapeutic communication in a clinical setting. His pet-oriented psychotherapy work with his dog Jingles was published in 1962 in the journal *Mental Hygiene*.[54] He published his landmark book, *Pet-Oriented Child Psychotherapy*, in 1969 explaining how the pet serves as a transitional object in facilitating the client-therapist relationship.[55] However, Levinson was ridiculed and mocked in 1961 when he presented his findings at the annual convention of the American Psychological Association. It would ultimately be the collaborative work of Jofi and Freud that would propel Levinson's theory on pet-oriented psychotherapy into legitimacy in the skeptical 1960s psychological community.[56]

Today, animal-assisted interventions mirror Jofi's collaboration with Freud. In 2005, M. L. Glucksman wrote in the *Journal of the American Academy of Psychoanalysis and Dynamic Psychiatry* that Joe, a Labrador retriever, accompanied an analyst in the consulting room and that patients found the dog soothing and reassuring. Beyond the comfort, he reported that the dog functioned as a transitional object and transference displacement and occasionally was incorporated into the patient's defenses and resistance. Joe facilitated aspects of the therapeutic process such as exploring feelings and working through them and understanding and interpreting the session content. Glucksman described the most important role of the dog in the consulting room as being a "nonjudgmental, loyal and supportive co-therapist."[57] Fine has reported that an American Psychiatric Association survey showed that 21 percent of members used animals or animal content in therapy.[58] Their clinical use of animals was mostly symbolic; the clinicians often incorporated animal content to develop underlying themes or interpretations of the patient's clinical material.

Perhaps Jofi's most significant legacy was that she was the first therapy dog pioneer to break the "glass ceiling" of psychoanalytical partnership with a therapy dog. Her presence in the consulting room of the father of psychoanalysis provided the foundation for the legitimacy of the benefit of animals in mental health work. Although Freud did not explain in his own writings how Jofi helped the therapeutic process, his colleagues and patients observed

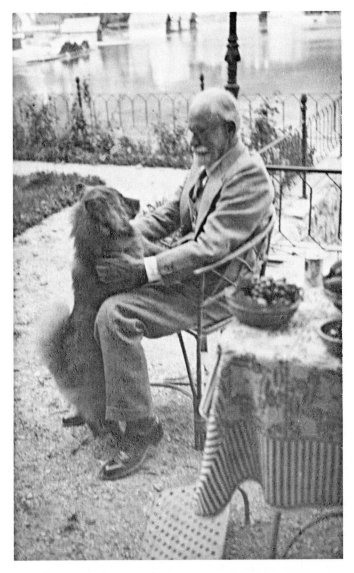

Sigmund Freud and Jofi, 1937 (Freud Museum, London).

that he seemed to experience and respect what she could teach. It would be up to future scientists, philosophers, and students of the human-animal bond to study why and how the human-animal bond functions in a therapeutic setting. However, it wasn't until decades later in 1960 that Boris Levinson and his dog Jingles would be the next pioneering partners in the psychiatric consulting room, this time with children.

3

Cap and Florence Nightingale

The old shepherd's eyes filled with tears as he looked at his beloved sheepdog and explained his plan to 17-year-old Florence Nightingale. "I'm going to hang him."

"Oh, Roger, what has dear old Cap done?"

"He has done nothing, but he will never be any use to me, and I cannot afford to keep him." Roger drove his spade into the ground and concentrated on it to keep from crying.

"Two boys threw a stone at Cap yesterday, and the stone hit his leg. I am afraid that the stone broke Cap's leg."

Florence Nightingale knew that even a shepherd's favorite sheepdog had to be able to work. A broken leg in a working dog could end his herding days, and Cap had not been able to walk since he was hurt.

Florence Nightingale and the local church vicar often rode together in the woods near her country home in Embry. Earlier today, they had interrupted their ride when they saw Roger, the shepherd who lived in one of the cottages in the woods on the downs. Florence and the vicar had noticed something unusual when they stopped to talk with Roger as he tended his sheep. He was finishing up for the day, but noisy sheep were scattered in all directions and Cap, Roger's sheepdog, was nowhere in sight. Cap had a reputation as an excellent sheepdog, and he knew his job well. He was usually with Roger. Since Roger had no wife or children, Cap served as both a work partner and a companion to the shepherd.

The vicar suggested to Florence that Cap's leg might not actually be broken since it would take a hard blow to break the bone of a dog like Cap. Before they started home, Florence and the vicar decided to go to the shepherd's cabin to see Cap's injury for themselves. They planned to find the dog and look at Cap's leg to see if anything could be done.

When they arrived at the cottage, they discovered Cap lying on the bare brick floor, under the table. The usually energetic sheepdog whined, whimpered, and struggled to move. When Florence called "Cap," his tail wagged, and he crept *out from under the table just far enough to greet them. As she kneeled down on the mud floor, Florence saw the dog wince and heard another whine, softer now, as if he did not want to complain.*

They needed to look at that leg. Florence patted Cap's head as he lay at her feet. As she took one of his paws in her hand, she softly talked to Cap as the vicar carefully examined the injury. Cap moaned, winced, and licked the two gentle hands that touched him.

The vicar declared it was a bad bruise, but no bones were broken. He thought resting the leg might help. Florence looked at the dog; he was still whining softly and was barely able to move. She wondered if they could do something to help the pain. She decided to try hot water to foment the wound to ease the pain.[1] Florence found an old flannel petticoat, ripped it into strips, soaked the strips in warm water, and wrung them out. Then she tenderly applied them to the dog.

As Florence and the vicar started home, they met Roger. He was carrying a piece of rope. Florence told him that Cap's leg was not broken and he would not have to hang him. No rope was needed—at least not today.

Florence visited Cap the next day. The swelling in his leg was down. She bathed the wound again. In a few days, Cap was back on duty working his sheep. The next time Florence met Cap and Roger together on the downs, Roger thanked her: "But for you, I would have hung the best dog I ever had."[2]

Cap had met the girl who would become the health care heroine of England, and Florence Nightingale had successfully treated her first patient.

The story of Cap and Florence Nightingale appeared in most reports of Nightingale's childhood[3] and became an enduring part of her heroic narrative.[4] Some proposed that the early experience mending a sheepdog's leg was part of the root cause for Florence's later vision and call to a life of service. The Cap story appears in various versions in reports of the life of Florence Nightingale and but contained the same basic facts and was handed down in accounts of Florence Nightingale's life and work.

Was Cap's influence on Nightingale myth, mysticism, or just a good dog story? What role could a sheepdog with an injured leg play in the life and calling of this iconoclastic legend? Most biographers of Nightingale agree that the healing event of Cap on the hillside actually occurred. The story of Cap was an appealing part of the legend that created the admiration for Nightingale and contributed to the strength of persuasion that propelled Nightingale's causes. In his comprehensive 2008 biography, *Florence Nightingale: The Making of an Icon*, Mark Bostridge meticulously traced the life and myth of Nightingale and pointed out that while the relative significance of Cap in the Nightingale story may be exaggerated, it seems to have a basis in fact and provenance.[5] A key theme of Bostridge's biography is the way in which Nightingale's life is characterized by the constant interaction of life and myth.[6] It is at this intersection that Cap becomes part of the Nightingale story.

The "Redundant" Woman

Florence Nightingale was unexpected—an unmarried, independent woman in Victorian England who said she had a direct calling from God. She pursued an independent life, and she learned how to create that life on her own terms. Florence Nightingale's image and legend is of a kind and caring ministering angel of mercy and the founder of modern nursing—the "Lady with the Lamp." The Nightingale reality is more complex—and more intriguing because a sheepdog may have played a pivotal role.

Florence Nightingale was a woman of contradictions—part legend, part visionary, part social reformer, part scientist, and part pioneer. She was a gentle spirit of healing who was also a bold thinker and reformer who said and wrote exactly what she thought. Nightingale was a woman of great compassion, tenderness, strength, boldness, and mystery. In Victorian England, she needed to be all these things to advance desperately needed improvements in health care.

Nightingale inspired admiration and controversy in Victorian England and continues to do so today. The Lady with the Lamp had numerous critics and detractors along with admirers and advocates. She engendered both sentimental appeal and harsh condemnation. As a young, unmarried Victorian woman, she was equipped with education, and it was not surprising she might seek a different path than most young women.[7] She would become a woman leading male doctors and political leaders and was a radical thinker. She was a heroine who fought disease and social injustice and advanced the nursing profession into an acceptable role for educated women.

Her accomplishments extended beyond her best-known work to improve conditions of the military in the Crimean War. She improved health care, hospital organization, and sanitary conditions, advanced the cause of women, and made significant contributions to the measurement of health care outcomes and statistics. The fact that she lived and worked in seclusion after her return as a hero of the Crimea added to the mystery and speculation that surrounds her legacy and life.[8]

An animal lover from her childhood, Nightingale, was an early advocate of animal-assisted therapy. In Notes on Nursing, her classic treatise on nursing, she outlined basic concepts of care of the sick and nursing practice and wrote, "A small pet animal is often an excellent companion for the sick, for long chronic cases especially. A bird in a cage is sometimes the only pleasure of an invalid confined to years to the same room. If he can feed and clean the animal himself, he should be encouraged to do so."[9]

Analysis of Nightingale's myth and contributions are as varied as her biographers, but her contributions to nursing and health care are undisputed.[10] Her legend as a pioneer of health care and founder of modern nursing endures in spite of several publications that challenged her image and accomplishments.[11]

The romanticized, oversimplified versions of Florence Nightingale's life and achievements obscure her more complicated identity as a woman who could be harsh and blunt if that's what was needed to effect change. In 1918, British writer Lytton Strachey published his book *Eminent Victorians* that featured biographies of four famous Victorians as a commentary on Victorian life. He suggested Nightingale's "vision and the myth was one thing, the reality was different."[12] Strachey wrote that Nightingale was direct in her communication, especially with officials who needed to change, and that Nightingale was "not one to mince words." Strachey described her "irresistible authority" and claimed, "Her sarcasm searched the ranks of the officials with the deadly and unsparing precision of a machine gun."[13]

Bostridge suggested that her legend romanticized and possibly obscured the real woman who was often complex and contradictory. He proposed that she knew how to publicize her name and her cause to advance them. Bostridge also suggested that Nightingale was also a caring, complicated iconoclast who may have constructed her own persona to promote her objectives and to improve health care.[14]

We are left with an intriguing question: Was Cap just part of the Nightingale myth or was he indeed her inspiration?

Florence Nightingale grew up in Victorian England when women were expected to do one thing: enter into a good marriage and raise a family. She was the second daughter of well-to-do English parents. Her mother was socially active in Victorian society, and her father had inherited wealth. She was born in 1820 and named after Florence, Italy, the city of her birth. The Nightingale family returned to England from Florence after a leisurely continental tour and settled in a family home, Lea Hall, which was replaced by a larger house, Lea Hurst. In 1825 Nightingale's father purchased Embley Park, a 4,000-acre estate on the edge of the New Forest, Hampshire, and when Florence was five the Nightingale family alternated between the two estates. She grew up in great wealth and luxury.

Florence's early life as a daughter of privilege provided her with advantages, one of which was an education in math, foreign languages, and literature. She was educated at home by her father, William Edward Nightingale, who was a student of the classics and had studied at Trinity College in Cambridge. Young Victorian women did not attend university. Her father believed young women should be educated, and unlike most young women, Florence received a rich and robust education, and she learned how to think for herself.

As a young woman, Nightingale enjoyed an active social life in addition to being contemplative. Tall and graceful, she was elegant rather than beautiful, with straight hair and brown eyes. She was described as fun. She was reported to have a talent for mimicry, which provided much delight. She had opportunities to meet others and was said to be found attractive to both men and women.[15] Although she had several marriage proposals, Nightingale remained unmarried throughout her life. She believed a husband would interfere with her career aspirations.

In Nightingale's era, women who failed to find a suitable husband and raise a family were labeled as "the odd woman" or "the redundant woman." In fact, single women who remained unmarried were viewed as a growing social problem in Victorian England. In 1869, William Rathbone Greg published an essay, "Why are Women Redundant," expressing concern for the high number of superfluous women in Victorian England who remained unmarried in the 19th century.[16] Greg proposed massive shipments of unmarried women to the British colonies, where single men were plentiful and supposedly eager for wives. As it turned out, young, educated women in England did not find Greg's proposal very attractive and did not rush to take advantage of the offer.

Women were beginning to question paternalistic Victorian society and the ideal of the traditional Victorian marriage. At the time, men were considered the only ones who took action. Women were the nurturers, caretakers, wives, and mothers. The defined roles of women and men were separate and rigid.

As she came of age amidst this Victorian mindset, Florence Nightingale had no intention of marrying or being in any way superfluous or redundant. She may not have had a plan, but Florence Nightingale had plenty of dreams. Many suggested that those dreams had been inspired by Cap, a shepherd's sheepdog.

The Dream Begins

Having treated Cap as her first patient, young Miss Nightingale went on to live her life as a young Victorian woman, although her life was anything but ordinary. Higher education for women was not expected for young Victorian women who were considered successful if they found a husband and took care of him and their home and family, but Florence studied Greek, Latin, music, and English literature. She read contemporary poets and enjoyed adventure stories. She became fluent in French, German, and Italian.[17] At age 20, Florence asked to study mathematics and was eventually allowed to study mathematics under a tutor.[18] As she grew up, she continued to show great care for animals and those who were needy or ill.

In 1837, when she was 17 years old, she reported that she had received a direct call from God. She struggled with the path that calling should take, and her quest to find her real purpose would not be quick or easy. She spent years dreaming about what she should do to answer God's call. Her personal writing indicated that these dreams were a source of considerable anxiety. The amount of time she spent on her dreaming was so troubling to Florence that she viewed her dreams as an affliction.[19] She reportedly also had periods of despair.

She struggled against the conventional life of Victorian women and longed for a profession or a trade to fill her with purpose. She would struggle with her path for 16 years before beginning a pioneering career that would transform health care and society. Florence experienced years of conflict at home before she was allowed to free herself to pursue her dream.

She was determined to find her way out of the life of middle-aged Victoria women, which she saw as one of idleness and waste. In 1852 she wrote a political essay, "Cassandra," as an angry outcry against the forced idleness of Victorian women. It was a work that showed her despair and anger at women's position and was a protest against the powerlessness of women. The writing of "Cassandra" seemed to move Florence from despair into rebellion.[20]

The seeds of restlessness had been planted in Florence early in her history. The Nightingale family had a tradition of working for social reform. Her maternal grandfather had been an anti-slavery campaigner. Her strong religious background gave her a sense of moral duty to help the poor and disadvantaged.[21]

Young Nightingale prepared for her future, although she was still unsure what form it might take. She studied hospital reports and learned about social reform. She said she received two more calls from God and finally, in 1853, she gained freedom from her family to pursue her true vocation, of which she was now sure.[22]

She came to believe that nursing was her God-inspired vocation. She had endured despair and confusion, at times agonized, and wished her day-dreaming of a life of purpose and accomplishment would cease altogether.[23] There were some who speculated that her early experience ministering to Cap, the shepherd's sheepdog, had inspired her first calling to nursing and caring for the ill.

Her choice of nursing as a calling, however inspired, was not popular with her well-to-do parents and was not encouraged by them. The appropriate role for a daughter of a wealthy Victorian family was to find a husband after a proper series of dances, social events, and introductions to society. Florence's female cousin and sister dutifully followed this path.

Nursing was a dubious calling for any respectable young woman. Nurses were viewed as disreputable, immoral, dirty, uneducated, and involved in various questionable pursuits. The morals and motives of any unmarried Victorian woman who chose a career that included contact with naked bodies, both male, and female, were questionable.[24] Nursing's image was sometimes associated with prostitution or inappropriate relationships with patients. Many parents even today might think twice before funding such a career pursuit. However, as many a parent of a determined young person has learned, children have their own plans, and Florence Nightingale was determined. Florence would follow her calling despite her parents' opposition.

Nightingale continued to prepare herself for a future of service. She struggled to pursue her dream; she studied histories, visited nursing institutions, and convinced her parents to allow her to complete 3-month training at a hospital and school in Dusseldorf, the Kaiserworth Deaconess Institute. It was to be a significant event in her life. For her, the pursuit of a nursing vocation was to become much more than nursing.

Fortunately, Florence Nightingale, unlike many other Victorian women, had the means to make a choice.[25] However, her calling and her departure from the expected role of the Victorian woman would prove a challenge and a rocky path for the rest of her life.

Luckily, Nightingale developed a talent for being in the right place at the right time.[26] When Florence was 33 years, the opportunity presented itself, and she became the superintendent of the Hospital for Sick Governesses in Harley, where she served from August 1853 to October 1854.[27] Her father provided her an annuity to allow her to support herself to take the position at the small hospital. She organized supplies, moved the dispensary in-house, reduced staff, reduced costs, and assisted with minor surgeries.[28] The assignment formed the foundation of her nursing career.

She would later set up a nursing school to improve opportunities for women in nursing, believing that an obstacle to women entering the profession was the impression that they would be exposed to various dangers of immorality and especially alcohol and drinking.[29] It was an impression that was valid until Nightingale arrived to change nursing forever.

While she was at Harley, another opportunity appeared. She was called to assist at the military hospitals in the Crimean War. France, Britain, Russia, and Turkey were competing for territory in the Middle East, and religious differences and the importance of the area created war. In March 1854, reports of military hospitals' lack of medical supplies and poor conditions created a public outcry. Badly needed sheets sent by steamship arrived in the wrong place.[30] Wounded men were shipped in batches of 200 across the Black Sea to Scutari. The journey took about 3 weeks for a 3-day trip. There were little supplies or food or blankets, and inadequate sanitary conditions. For months the average death rate was 74 per 1,000. Corpses were shot out into the water.[31] When the wounded arrived at the hospital in Scutari, conditions were deplorable.

Nightingale was ready. She already had experience in supply management and improving hospital services and had studied hospital operations. Florence Nightingale was dispatched to oversee the introduction of her trained female nurses into the military hospitals in Crimea. In 1854, she led the first team of 38 British nurses to war in the Crimea.[32] They organized wards, brought supplies, arranged beds, and improved sanitary conditions.

Florence Nightingale was strict, determined, outspoken, smart, and organized. She studied processes to find out how to make them better. She gathered data and measured outcomes. She was blunt, direct, and tolerated no inefficiency or lack of kindness. Her habit of rounding at night to check on conditions and the sick earned her the name of the "Lady with the Lamp." She had come to hell and was going to transform it into a clean, orderly place of healing. She returned to England as a heroine.

No Place for a Lady

Nightingale's contribution in the Crimea was only the beginning of her pioneering work. Health care in England desperately needed reforms. Nursing required transformation into an occupation that could attract educated women who, although they may have been raised in the drawing rooms of respectable Victorian society, they yearned to do more than needlework.

However, Victorian hospitals were no place for a well-bred, educated Victorian woman. The odor of filth and the squalor were so bad that visitors were often overcome by nausea. Wood floors were saturated with organic material and waste that when washed smelled worse than before; walls and ceilings were saturated with contaminated material, and a single fire supplied the heat. The smell became sickening as the walls might ooze steamed moisture, and small vegetation appeared. Men who washed the walls, which was done with lime, frequently became seriously ill.

Patients came in dirty and stayed dirty. Liquor was shared among patients and staff, and police sometimes had to be called in to restore order. Beds were arranged less than 2 feet apart, with 50 or 60 people crammed in a room. Patients came from slums and tenements and brought cholera, which spread quickly with unsanitary practices and close quarters. Nurse slept, ate, and worked in the ward. Nurses often alternated their nursing duties with prostitution. Many slept on the wards, sometimes with male patients on the male wards. Drastic understaffing meant that a single night nurse might have charge of four wards. Privacy was impossible.[33]

Health care reform was a huge challenge. The outside environment from which the patients came was no better. Victorian London itself was filthy. Choking sooty fog challenged breathing. The Thames River ran thick with sewage, and the streets were covered with mud that was really horse dung. With tens of thousands of horses, dung was a fact of life. Boys would be hired to dodge in between the horse traffic to catch the manure as soon as it hit the already dirty street.

The stench rose from cesspools and blocked drains. Urine soaked the streets. The smell of ammonia was overpowering, and storekeepers said the ammonia was destroying the shop fronts. Lee Jackson, who wrote about the battle against these conditions in his book *Dirty Old London: The Victorian Fight Against Filth*,[34] commented: "The idea that ... the stench is coming into the house, seeping through the house and possibly bringing in diseases like cholera or typhoid ... is actually one of the great driving forces of sanitary reform in the 19th century."[35]

The Victorians lived with surges of waste, dump, and smell. If you were poor, your water came from a standpipe provided by your property owner, and that water might be turned on for one or two hours a week. If you wanted to wash, no other routes existed; working men might use rivers, canals, or lakes to bathe. This was the environment in which Nightingale found herself as she set out to reform the conditions in civilian hospitals.

The scandal of the conditions at Scutari and Nightingale's pioneering work led the Royal Commission to investigate the conditions and care in military hospitals, which led to other improvements in health care in the civilian population. Donations then poured into the Nightingale Fund, which supported the reform of civilian hospitals in the post-war period and hygienic practices. Nightingale was now in a position to change health care. Her dream had begun.

Nightingale knew she needed more than the power of the sweet Lady with the Lamp. She understood that measurement mattered. Nightingale utilized statistics and data to communicate the need for change in health care. Change in long-held practices often comes slowly; people and organizations need to be convinced to change when they have done things a certain way for years.

Florence Nightingale had a powerful tool. She had data and knew how to use it. She used statistics to show that more men were dying from unhygienic conditions and the diseases they caused than from the war.[36] She determined that high death rates such as those that occurred in the army hospitals should never happen again and created a 900-page analysis of root causes for the high death rate. She succeeded in getting a royal commission to investigate and publicly report its findings. In 1858, Nightingale presented a "Paper on the Sanitary Conditions in the Construction of Hospital Wards" at the Liverpool meeting of the Association of Social Scientists. She provided notes on defects she had observed based on her own experience. Her improvements in the British army in India demonstrated that bad drainage, contaminated water, and poor hygiene affected health outcomes. She demonstrated with data that the health of the army and that of civilians were connected, and she worked to improve the health of India as a whole. She demonstrated a way to measure health outcomes using risk-adjusted comparative data, wherein the data were adjusted based on the diseases and risks of different groups of patients.[37] Nightingale showed that current hospital statistics and measures of mortality were not adequate measures of the sanitary conditions of hospitals. She explained the principles of measurement to the committee: "If the function of a hospital were to kill the sick, statistical comparisons of this nature would be admissible."[38] It's not likely her audience appreciated Nightingale's talent for stating the obvious.

Nevertheless, Florence Nightingale was the first woman elected to the Royal Statistical Society in 1909.[39] Nightingale went on to identify the need for improvement in inadequate ventilation, overcrowding, defects in construction, and deficiency of light, and she laid out specific recommendations to accomplish them. She emphasized that the most pressing problem was the need to find trained and qualified nurses.

Florence Nightingale's influence on nursing alone would have transformed health care. She established nursing as an acceptable profession. She successfully introduced female nurses into the military, established hygienic practices in hospitals, and was the heroine of the Crimean War. She improved hospital ward design, nutrition, care of beds and bedding in the sick room, and cleanliness of the room, walls, and floors. She included notes on personal cleanliness and its impact on infection, offered her opinions on excess "chattering" to the sick, and suggested ways to communicate with a sick person that would be the most helpful to healing. She cautioned nurses to beware of any visitors who tell a sick person "that he has nothing the matter with him."[40]

She wrote of the need to create a healthy environment at home. Her proposed healthy environment was comprehensive in scope. It included air, water, drainage, cleanliness, ventilation of sick rooms, and noise; appropriate dress for those nursing the sick; behavior when visiting the sick; the interconnectedness of body and mind; and the therapeutic effect of music, flowers, air, and light. She advocated a healthy diet, pioneered midwifery, and used statistics to measure outcomes and prove the need for improvement. *Notes on Nursing* provided instruction on the observation of the patient and sanitary nursing procedures that are still valued today. She professed a nursing principle that endures today: What nursing must do is to "put the patient in the best condition for nature to act upon him."[41] The Nightingale School was established in 1860, and then schools were started in the United States, Australia, and around the world.

Her accomplishments reached far beyond nursing. She became a pioneering health reformer, a system thinker, and author. She wrote more than 10,000 letters and reports, books, articles, and letters to the editor and other documents that appear in more than 200 archives worldwide.[42] Lynn McDonald compiled these in the *Collected Works of Florence Nightingale*. The last of the 16 volumes was published in 2013, and the series has more than 14,000 pages. Florence Nightingale inspired the founding of the International Red Cross. Nightingale met and corresponded with Queen Victoria over a span of 30 years.

Although she was confined to her bed for decades for what was believed to be brucellosis, Florence Nightingale remained a driving force in social reform and health care. Many of her most significant achievements occurred after her return from the Crimea.[43] She was a woman who learned how to advance what she believed in. Her tools were data, her own persona, her strength of faith, and her compelling personal narrative mixed with the ability to navigate the political reality that she was a strong, determined woman pioneering social change in a world where such an unmarried woman was considered redundant.

Volumes have been written about the legend, life, and work of Florence Nightingale. Personal and historical narratives are subject to interpretation. Some celebrate her, and some cynics attempt to debunk the myths.[44] She was a pioneer, and pioneers travel their journey uphill much of the time. She was denounced for her pioneering analysis of postnatal mortality. The famous story of Florence and Cap notwithstanding, an anonymous note in a leading medical journal of her time disputed her findings and called it a failure of her "kind womanly heart."[45]

Florence Nightingale knew how to make things happen. If she wanted something done, she went about it in whatever way she could. Nightingale's was an age where femininity was revered, and its essence was to serve others. Nightingale's more gentle myth and persona allowed her to be given hero status because she sacrificed and cared for others—even a poor sheepdog. For the rest of her life, she would remain a figure who inspired legend, inspiration, and controversy.

Cap: Mysticism or Just a Dog Story?

While Nightingale and her life have inspired different interpretations, the significance of Cap, a simple injured sheepdog, to this pioneering Nightingale journey has invited almost as much speculation. Did a sheepdog influence the dream and the woman and move the destiny and legacy of Florence Nightingale forward? Some said her early experience healing the sheepdog was the defining moment in that call to service. Others held that her love of animals blended into her love of medicine and nursing and that "her kindness on the hillside was destined to be repeated in the eyes of the suffering men as she bent over them in Scutari."[46]

Cap was both ordinary and extraordinary. He was a typical local sheepdog with normal sheepdog duties. He had a reputation for being both a great herder and clever. Roger called Cap "the best dog I ever had." Cap was described as a "very sensible dog," and it was reported that "people used to say Cap could do everything but speak."[47]

By most reports, Cap kept the sheep in proper order and provided excellent service to his master. On the day Cap was hit by a stone thrown by boys, neither Cap nor Roger could have imagined that Cap's reputation was about to expand far beyond his sheep-herding days.

Cap is frequently described in historical accounts as a shepherd's collie, or farm collie, an informal class of collie-like herding dogs. He was probably a collie-like dog whose primary function was herding of farm animals or performing farm work. A sheepdog such as Cap might be descended from any of the collie breeds. Today many breeds function as herding dogs, and the American Working Collie Association registers farm collies based on working ability rather than breed.[48] The farm collie/sheepdog is an active dog that requires mental stimulation, challenge, and activity, and the future of a dog with a broken leg or an unhealed wound that could not work would look grim indeed to a shepherd.

Cap was valuable to Roger as both companion and colleague for working and herding the flock. Roger would have invested considerable time in training his work partner, and the dog would have great value to the shepherd. The primary purpose of herding dogs is to move their flock. Usually, herding dogs are trained to respond to a command or whistle. Herding dogs work in a variety of ways. Herding is based on modified natural prey behavior with training. Some nip at the heel of animals and are called heelers. Others stare down the animal and are known as headers. Border collies usually are headers. They consistently go to the front of the group of animals to turn or stop an animal's movement. Heeler or driving dogs keep animals moving forward. Some breeds work more independently and are called tending dogs, who act as sort of a living fence while guiding large flocks of sheep to graze while preventing them from wandering and are able to gather large groups of sheep.

It was not unusual for a sheepdog to experience an injury. Farm dogs are prone to injuries as part of the job—with broken legs or bruising from getting caught in fences or in barbed wire or from falling—and a shepherd's knowledge of first aid can be helpful.[49] Livestock management and animal husbandry were undergoing changes in the Victorian era. There was no refrigeration, so slaughtering had to be done close to cities, and herds of cattle, sheep, and pigs might need to be driven through the streets. Sheep were also viewed as a symbol of the lower class in a society where wealth and class status were paramount.[50]

A sheepdog not only represented a farmer's livelihood but was often close to his heart. Saving Cap to herd another day was a significant contribution by young Florence to Roger's life and well-being.

As extraordinary a dog as Cap was in his duties on the farm, could an early experience with such a sheepdog inspire someone to find his or her own life purpose? For some, Florence Nightingale was not just a visionary and a healer, but a mystic.[51] Cap was her first patient, but the incident has also been interpreted as an indication of her early calling and affinity to help hurt creatures. It is not difficult to imagine that Nightingale herself might have considered the healing of Cap and her vision part of the mystical experience of being close to God and learning his purpose for her life.

Vicar Giffard, who had accompanied Florence that day on the farm, provided a firsthand account of the event and a simple interpretation. He interpreted Florence's healing of Cap as an indication that people who are kind to animals will be kind to people. The event showed the concern for others that would characterize her life's work.[52]

Others extended the meaning of Cap's story further, linking her early experience healing a sheepdog to her later calling from God and vision. Florence Nightingale believed she received a direct call from God.[53] In 1874, she wrote that she had heard inner voices four times in her life: in 1837,[54] 1853, 1854, and 1861.[55] Her life was based on a reaction to that call.

Barbara Dossey, Ph.D., a nurse, and Florence Nightingale scholar, has written extensively on Nightingale as a visionary and mystic. Dossey defined mysticism as a way of life that flows from a direct experience of God, however conceived, and that "a mystic is one who, to a greater or lesser degree, has the experience of being at one with God."[56] Florence Nightingale experienced her call from God as a call to serve those in need. Dossey suggested that Florence Nightingale's mysticism moved the nursing profession towards an integrative approach to political, moral, aesthetic, and spiritual aspects of care for their patients.[57] Evelyn Underhill, one of the most respected authorities on Western mysticism in the 20th century, described Nightingale as "one of the greatest and most balanced contemplatives of the nineteenth century."[58] The source of her strength, vision, and guidance was a deep sense of unity with God, which is the hallmark of the mystical tradition in all the world's great religions. Nightingale believed that every person who was drawn to ease the pain and suffering of another is an instrument of genuine healing.

When her legacy and accomplishments are considered, they must be viewed in light of her foundation in mysticism.[59]

A dog can often have symbolic meaning in the course of a person's life or future events. Stanley Coren who writes extensively on the history and mental abilities of dogs, looked at this event in the context of Florence's later dream or calling.[60] He discussed dogs as "sentinels and symbols" in which "the actions of a single dog changed the life of a single human, who in turn went on to shape human history."[61] Coren noted that the Cap incident occurred in February of 1837 when Florence was 17. Coren also cited reports extracted from her diaries[62] that the very next night, February 7, 1837, Florence Nightingale had her first dream or vision informing her that she had a mission. Coren countered the argument by admitting that perhaps it was a result of knowing she had helped a living thing that had been suffering that caused Nightingale to believe that the whole incident was a sign from God that she should devote her life to helping others.[63]

Mystical experience or not, Cap's story was transformational in several ways. The social society and health care system of Florence Nightingale's day needed transformation, and she knew it. Changemakers usually understand that the key to harnessing the power of an identified community is the power of shared narrative through metaphors, symbols, and images. Stories are transformational. Nightingale needed a powerful but sympathetic narrative. Florence Nightingale needed a good story.

Societies share stories to communicate with each other and create meaning. When a story shows kindness, healing, or hope in the face of cruelty or suffering, the abstract concepts of compassion and empathy are powerfully communicated in a way we understand. A transformational tale moves storyteller and listener both to create their own meaning.[64] Health care and improvement in health care often unfold in stories of modern medicine and depend on the listening, telling, interpreting, and acting on narrative accounts and stories.[65]

For Nightingale working in Victorian England, a shared narrative was needed to create an identified community to transform nursing into a trusted profession. She needed to be seen as a respectable, kind, and compassionate figure that represented the profession well. That effort succeeded. A 2016 Gallop poll showed that nurses were the most trusted profession for the fifth straight year.[66]

Nightingale's personal story had played a role in her accomplishments— with her intelligence, her many contributions, and her scientific, political, and practical understanding of the environment. She contributed to the transformation of health care on many fronts: nursing, nursing administration, nursing ethics, nursing education, hospital operations, hygiene and sanitation, home care, outcomes measurement, statistics, holistic/integrative care, and social reforms. Beyond that, she was an early advocate for animal-assisted therapy and the healing power of pets.

Was Cap just part of the Nightingale myth or was he a true pioneer dog and her inspiration? Mystical experience or transformational story, Cap was a Dog Pioneer who served as a symbol.

Cap's Legacy: What If?

What if the shepherd had hung poor Cap before Florence Nightingale intervened? One approach to evaluating the significance of historical events is used by historians who employ a technique called counterfactual reasoning, in which past events are analyzed by asking what would have occurred in history if the particular event had not occurred.[67] As Gavriel D. Rosenfeld pointed out in his 2014 blog, "Counterfactual Canines: How Would History Have Been Different Without Dogs," there is danger in attributing small events to significant changes in the future of a person.[68]

However, this approach leads to several possibilities. What if Florence Nightingale had not met Roger the shepherd that day on the meadow? What if the boys had not thrown a rock that injured poor Cap? Florence Nightingale may have still had her vision or calling from God, and she still may have pursued her life of accomplishment. We are left with even more intriguing questions. Did Cap inspire Florence Nightingale's calling, or was he a result of it? What did Nightingale herself believe about the impact of her first patient on her life? What difference did the story of Cap make in the Nightingale story?

The most straightforward interpretation of Cap's story may be that of the vicar who accompanied her on her ride that day and who helped her repair Cap's wounded leg: The action was an indicator of the character of the woman who would do so much good to help people. This line of thinking helps establish Florence Nightingale as a beacon of gentleness and compassion and an exemplary example of Victorian womanhood. The story of the healing of Cap by Florence Nightingale was likely to affect Victorian England's view of her as a gentle heroine. It contributed to the myth and legend of the Lady with the Lamp—a story needed to advance her cause at a time when conflict and barriers confronted a determined, brash, unmarried reformer.

It is probably safe to assume Nightingale was aware of the proliferation of the Cap story. Bostridge noted that the vicar published his story about Cap with Nightingale's knowledge and permission.[69]

The leader of a reform movement needs to be able to identify with the community it seeks to change. Florence Nightingale knew, in her Victorian world, that nursing and nurses had an image problem. A respectable, unmarried woman who was seen as gentle, kind, and fond of animals who also chose nursing as a profession would be helpful to advance the nursing profession in a medical world managed by male culture. Nightingale needed to serve as a role model for the Victorian women she wanted to recruit into nursing.

Can a dog inspire a mystical vision? Dr. Diane Pomerance, a pet grief recovery specialist and author, wrote about the interconnectedness of animals and spirituality and explained that they can teach us lessons about our own spirituality and connect us to the world of nature.[70] Through the existence of animals and being close to them, we can recognize the spiritual gifts that

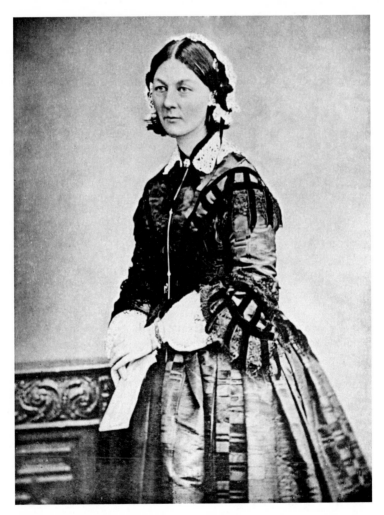

Florence Nightingale, between 1860 and 1870 (Library of Congress).

life has to offer. In their book, *Angel Dogs, Divine Messengers of Love*, Allen and Linda Anderson wrote that the spiritual nature of dogs is rarely written about, perhaps due to fears of further anthropomorphizing or becoming overly sentimental about dogs. The Andersons shared stories of those who have experienced dogs as divine messengers.[71]

At its most expansive, the experience with Cap may have been the catalyst for a mystical experience for Nightingale, her call to a career of incredible service and accomplishments in health care and health care reform. Whether or not that occurred is a question that, like many transformational experiences with dogs and their connection to humans at pivotal moments, may not always need an answer or a proof of cause and effect. Dogs show us something we need to see.

We do know Cap was an essential part of Florence Nightingale's story. The power of that story created part of the myth that softened the persona of the bold, determined unmarried iconoclast for her Victorian audience. Who could resist someone whose first patient was an injured sheepdog and who, at an early age, knew what to do to save him?

Dogs often find humans just when we are most ready to see what they can show us—just when we are most ready to listen and learn. Perhaps this was true for Cap and Florence. Dogs teach us by showing, not informing. It is up to us to find meaning in their lessons. Perhaps Cap was the first to show Florence Nightingale a way to find the meaning and purpose she had so longed for. Cap appeared in her young life and became part of the myth, and together the story carried them both forward to change health care forever.

Myth, muse, or mystic, Cap helped develop the force that was the Lady with the Lamp. Today Nightingale is regarded as one of the most admired figures in the history of health care and is considered by some to be one of the most compassionate persons in history.[72]

Health care reform requires heroes, never more than today. The challenges are many: the stigma in using mental health services, infection control, fighting new diseases in poverty-stricken areas, recruitment of sufficient nurses, and measurement of relevant outcome data to drive evidence-based care, to name a few.

What if in treating Cap, Florence Nightingale first experienced the joy of helping and healing another living being? What if dogs were able to show us how to deliver comforting medicine and care where it was most needed, inspiring new pioneers to follow Nightingale's example?

What if we were all ready to watch and learn?

4

Togo and Balto:
Public Health Heroes

It's been snowing for an hour in New York, and the dog is already covered in ice. He stands on the rock in Central Park, in New York City, just west of East Drive and 67th Street. Blistering snow and wind slam the dog, but this husky has seen worse weather. Since 1925, this bronze sculpture of a hero dog has stood on the rock to honor Balto, the media darling of the 1925 serum run to save Nome. During a diphtheria epidemic, in a blinding blizzard, Balto led sled dog teams 675 miles to deliver the antitoxin to Nome. It was his first run as a lead dog, and Balto was the first dog to cross the finish line. An inscription below the statue of the big dog reads:

> *Dedicated to the indomitable spirit of the sled dogs that relayed antitoxin six hundred miles over rough ice, across treacherous waters, through Arctic blizzards from Nenana to the relief of stricken Nome in the winter of 1925. Endurance. Fidelity. Intelligence.[1]*

In another part of the city, the New York snow also falls on another dog. This dog stands on the Lower East Side of Manhattan, in small Seward Park on East Broadway. No plaque honors this statue of a small, unnamed husky who stands poised in full gallop. He, like Balto, is covered in ice today. On sunnier days, visitors to the park often note that his ears are shiny because children jump on his back and enjoy holding on to his ears.[2] This dog is Togo, the powerful lead sled dog of Leonhard Seppala, famous sled dog musher and an unsung hero. Some claim Togo, not Balto, was the dog who was the real hero of the serum run. Togo led the longest and most hazardous part of the round trip of the serum race, but Togo would never have the fame and celebrity claimed by Balto, who became a celebrity with a statue in Central Park.

As a killer disease stalked Nome, Alaska, in 1925, these two canine pioneers, each in his own way, showed America the power of human-animal collaboration in health care delivery. Theirs is a collective achievement of sled dogs' leadership, inspiration, and the triumph of teamwork.

Balto and Togo were dogs with different strengths and destinies, but in the winter of 1925, they had one common mission—to save Nome from a diphtheria epidemic. Togo was big and strong; Balto was small for his breed. Togo was an experienced lead dog; Balto had always been a follower and was a freight dog who had never led a team. Togo had the total respect and confidence of his trainer and handler, Leonhard Seppala; Balto never measured up to Seppala's expectations. Yet it was Balto who became a media star.

Their statues now sit in different parks. They ran their lives and races on separate trails and in different ways, but, at a pivotal moment in history, they ran one race, as public health servants to save a city.

Their achievement inspired efforts in disease prevention and public health care delivery in Alaska and the United States. The publicity of the collective accomplishments of Balto and Togo spurred an inoculation campaign that drastically reduced the threat of diphtheria.

American Legends

As diphtheria stalked Nome in the winter of 1925, the village was cold, isolated, ice-bound, and unprepared. A killer was advancing. The world watched and learned about leadership, teamwork, and the power of the human-animal bond as Togo and Balto, two canine pioneers, showed humans how to accomplish what seemed impossible: saving Nome from diphtheria, a dreaded disease known as the "strangler."[3] The dogs, the teams, and the serum race to save Nome would become an American legend.[4]

Through challenges of time, terrain, and the Alaska winter, sled dogs Togo and Balto led 20 men and 150 dogs in a unique cooperative interspecies effort to make history in public health and mass immunization. The teams of dogs, mushers, nurses, a doctor, and the people of Alaska collaborated to coordinate delivery of a life-saving serum.[5] Working in relays, the men and dogs delivered antitoxin to the village of Nome, completing the usual 674-mile trip in 127.5 hours. America watched, listened, and held its breath as 20 teams of dogs and men covered the brutal terrain for days on end in temperatures as low as 50 below zero to stop a catastrophic disease. Within days, the epidemic was contained.

Alaska in 1925: A Health Care Frontier

In 1925, Alaska was America's last frontier. It was an unforgiving environment with scarce health care resources and infrastructure. Alaskan territory covered an area one-fifth the size of the United States, and the extremes of terrain, climate, conditions, and culture affected both daily life and public health. While some Alaskans lived in cities, many resided in small rural communities isolated along navigational waterways or the seacoast.[6] The gold rush era closed just before World War I and, as a result, the population had doubled, dispersed through trails and roadhouses throughout the territory.[7]

Alaska's rugged trails were challenging in the best of weather. The cold could kill a man or a dog. In winter in Alaska, being cold could stop a man dead in his tracks. Nome winters were seven months long. In severe temperatures, a lost glove could mean losing a hand.[8]

Nome was remote. For nine months a year, it was practically unreachable. When the Bering Sea froze at the end of October, Nome was cut off from Seattle, the nearest port. In the 1920s, no air service existed except open cockpit airplanes. Flying an open-wing aircraft in Alaska's ice and the wind was treacherous. Pilots described the experience of operating in the white winter sky of the interior of Alaska with the snow on the ground as like "flying around inside a milk bottle."[9] The only way to reach Nome in winter was by a 325-mile train ride from Anchorage to Nenana, west of Fairbanks, and then by dogsled 674 miles more to Nome. The train station closest to Nome was icebound seven months of the year.

Dogsled teams and Alaska's mushers followed trails established over centuries by the Athabaskan Indians to cross the Interior Basin. They passed over mountains and rode across the ice along the coast of the Bering Sea. Then they struck across the ice of Norton Bay or went around to finally reach Nome, almost 700 miles from Nenana. With stopovers to rest dogs or change teams and drivers, the trip took between 25 and 30 days.[10]

Moving supplies when and where they are needed is essential for the delivery of health care. This requires transportation infrastructure. In Alaska, the cold and terrain dictated what was possible. Moving people and supplies and developing transportation capability was a critical factor in the development of Alaska. Navigational waterways defined the areas for development and provided access by dogsled.

Following the gold rush on the Seward Peninsula in the summer of 1900, Nome was a tent city with more than 20,000 men working the sands for gold. The discovery of gold in other parts of Alaska followed Nome's boom.[11] Eventually, expansion of railroad routes and air service would increase Alaska's ability to move health professionals and health supplies. The railroad was a boom to Alaska when the route from Seward to Fairbanks was completed in 1923. Reliable air access to remote areas was still evolving. Companies were beginning to secure contracts to deliver mail by plane. However, in the winter of 1925, neither railroad nor the coming air routes helped Alaska and its inhabitants escape disease.

Public health in Alaska was still frontier medicine. Small isolated communities lived along navigational routes. Before 1913, each settlement created its own public health rules and regulations, primarily concerned with quarantines, isolation of the sick, and burial of the dead. From 1867 to 1884, Alaska had no civil government infrastructure and was under the military jurisdiction of the army and navy.

After the gold rush, the population dispersed into small communities, and in 1912 Congress passed the second organic act creating a territorial government.[12] In 1913, the newly formed legislature of Alaska named the governor of Alaska as the commissioner of health. In 1915, the U.S. Department of Education assumed responsibility for the health of Alaskan natives, and the first federal hospital for treatment of Alaskan native populations was constructed in 1916.[13]

During World War I, there were few services and fewer practitioners, and when the flu epidemic hit Alaska in 1918, the Public Health Service assigned only 10 doctors.[14] In 1919, the Territorial Legislature created the office of the Commissioner of Health and appointed the first physician on a part-time basis. A series of laws became the authority and foundation for public health in Alaska. Territory-wide regulations were established for isolation and quarantine and provided for the organization of boards of health in various school districts in the territory. It was not until 20 years later that the passage of the Social Security Act would allocate funds for the development of Alaskan health services.[15]

Doctors and nurses in Alaska delivered care to remote areas under harsh conditions and often reached their patients by dogsled.[16] Later, many nurses flew by bush plane.[17] Alaska's hospitals consisted of six to 30 beds, were usually constructed of logs, and had a kitchen, a laundry, patient rooms, and rooms for staff to sleep. The one physician assigned was typically assigned to multiple coverage areas, and so nurses became critical to the delivery of health care in rural Alaska. The population, especially the native population, was widely dispersed. Some nurses moved from roles as hospital nurses to home care nurses, or so-called villager field nurses, and worked in brutal conditions to provide basic health services to isolated villages. Most nurses cooked and did the laundry and did 24-hour duty, for an annual average salary of $3,000.[18]

In 1925, Nome was a small law-abiding town of about 1,429 people.[19] Nome looked like most American towns, with the main street, a church, a post office, and a small hospital. Unlike most small towns, Nome had bone-chilling temperatures of 40 to 60 degrees below zero.

Dogs were essential to life in Nome. A good set of dogs meant survival. Dogs were work partners and a means of critical transportation, and they later became a source of recreation as dogsledding evolved as a sport.

Medical Team Brought Together by Fate

When the winter of 1925 began, Nome was cut off until the spring. Dr. Curtis Welch was acting assistant superintendent for the Public Health Service in charge of relief station 295 in Nome. As the only doctor for hundreds of miles, Welch was responsible for health care for Nome and the outlying communities.

Welch was a small man who looked slightly older than his 50 years; his blond hair was now white. He retained a hint of his Connecticut accent. Welch had a small staff of experienced nurses: Emily Morgan, Bertha Saville, and his wife, Lulu.

Curtis and Lulu Welch met while she was in nursing training at Los Angeles County Hospital. Lulu had wanted to be an actor but decided to pursue nursing. Curtis was a Yale Medical School graduate completing his internship at the hospital. They married and opened a hospital in Oakland, California, and worked side by side until Curtis met a colleague who wanted to give up his practice at a mining camp hospital in Council, Alaska, and they sailed from Seattle to Nome in 1907. After eight years, they moved from Council to Candle to manage Fairhaven Hospital, where they remained until the onset of World War I.

Curtis Welch wanted to be a soldier, and he intended to join the medical corps, but a replacement for him had to be found first. When a replacement was found, the Welches returned to Seattle. Dr. Welch waited to be called, but his military career was not to be. The armistice was signed before he was able to join the war effort. The Welches returned to Alaska for 10 more years.[20]

Nurse Emily Morgan was the head nurse at the two-story clapboard hospital. Morgan was a Kansas native who had been sent by the Red Cross to Alaska in 1923. A good head taller than Dr. Welch, she was good-natured, calm and easy to approach. Morgan had a nursing degree from Ellsworth Nurses Training School at Missouri Methodist Hospital in St. Joseph and had served as a nurse in World War I. After the war, she served as the first public health nurse in Wichita, Kansas. While serving as a school nurse, Morgan contracted diphtheria. She knew firsthand the symptoms of the terrible disease.[21] It was knowledge that was to come in handy as the winter of 1925 descended on Nome.

Nurse Bertha Saville usually accompanied Dr. Welch on his house calls. In the winter of 1925, she was set to leave her eight-year assignment as head nurse at the hospital for a position in the lower 48 states. Emily Morgan had been sent to replace her. Saville and Welch had an excellent clinical partnership. They had worked together for so long they anticipated each other's questions and thinking. Nurse Saville had another vital skill. She had experience working with native Eskimos and understood their culture and their lack of immunity from infectious diseases.[22] Every bit of her considerable nursing experience would be needed that winter.

On most days, the Welches' Nome medical practice was filled with the usual menu of small-town medicine: births, illness, injuries, death, and a variety of sicknesses. But in January 1925, an unusual threat loomed. Diphtheria was about to make a dramatic entry.

Fate had brought the small medical team together in the winter of 1925— Lulu Welch, a nurse who had planned to be an actor; Curtis Welch, a physician who had yearned to be a soldier; and two nurses who had come to the Alaska frontier to use their unique nursing experience. They found drama, adventure and a battle none of them could have predicted. Lulu found her drama, Curtis became a soldier in the fight of a deadly battle to save the people of Nome, and the nurses' unique experience and dedication would be put to their greatest use. The Nome medical team would also soon capture the world's attention.

The Strangling Angel

As the winter of 1925 descended on Nome, the residents of the isolated town were about to greet a visitor—the Strangling Angel of children.[23] Diphtheria had earned that name because those with the disease could feel like they were being strangled. Diphtheria is caused by a bacterium transmitted through close contact with infected individuals, usually by respiratory secretions. As the disease progresses, it produces thick secretions in the throat that make it difficult to breathe. Diphtheria can be fatal.[24] It was once a major cause of illness and death among children. Before treatment was available for diphtheria, almost half of those who contracted the disease died from it, but rates have dropped with the widespread use of vaccines.[25] The disease can be prevented by a vaccine or treated with an antitoxin.[26] The antitoxin needed in Nome could save lives if given in time, but it could not prevent diphtheria.[27]

In 1925, Alaskans feared epidemics. They had good reason. When the severe flu epidemic hit the Aleutian Islands in the 1900s, it killed the entire population of some villages. European and American explorers and traders had introduced new diseases for which native Alaskans had little or no natural immunity. In past epidemics, to combat the spread of the disease, some villages used armed guards. Cultural beliefs of native populations also affected acceptance of public health practice. Some residents believed that illnesses were caused by an angry supernatural spirit and were reluctant to accept treatment. Native Alaskans often had shamans who might be called upon to ease the wrath of spirits.[28]

In 1925, Alaskans were used to fighting cold and terrain. However, disease was still a severe threat to Nome, and Alaska still employed frontier medicine.[29] The challenges in fighting the spread of diseases like diphtheria included prompt identification of at-risk populations, surveillance for disease, diagnosis, prevention, treatment, and access to adequate supplies of vaccines and antitoxin.

The limited availability of medical personnel and resources and the lack of public health distribution channels in Alaska given the isolated and at-risk population compounded the challenges that confronted Nome in 1925. Missionaries and army and navy posts had provided much of the early health care.[30] Nurses also provided much of the care. Some communities organized Red Cross chapters. In the early 1900s, the Bureau of Education began to work to improve health care in isolated villages, and doctors and nurses aboard the bureau's supply ship would hold clinics during the summer months when the ship anchored. A nurse or doctor traveled by dogsled during the winter, and during the 1930s the staffing usually consisted of one doctor and two nurses at Barrow and a doctor at Nome.[31]

By January 20, 1925, Eskimo children in Nome were getting sick, and Curtis Welch's anxiety about possible diphtheria was rising. Dr. Welch and his nurses began to suspect diphtheria. Nurse Emily Morgan had been called to the home of a sick child and found her with a fever and symptoms of diphtheria; she took her suspicions back to Dr. Welch. He knew that with each day's incubation the disease could achieve epidemic proportions before antitoxin could be obtained. In the previous summer, Welch had checked his stock of diphtheria antitoxin; when he found it was outdated, he ordered a new supply, but it had not arrived. A second and then a third case were now suspected.

At first, diphtheria can look similar to several other diseases, and Dr. Welch was confronted with making a differential diagnosis—sorting through the diagnostic possibilities. In 1925, most doctors relied on signs and symptoms and if in doubt might take a throat culture that could determine the bacteria causing the symptoms. This took precious time. Welch had little experience with diphtheria.[32] In his 18 years of experience in the region, he had cases of tonsillitis and inflammation of the throat, but he had not seen a case of diphtheria.[33]

Welch had seen epidemics before. He had witnessed the flu pandemic of 1918 to 1919 and seen how an epidemic could wipe out villages and settlements with no disease resistance.[34] If diphtheria was about to strike, he knew it would spread rapidly and that it was deadly—especially for children. The Alaskan people had no immunity to the disease, and Welch recognized the need for antitoxin. He also was acutely aware that after the last ship left in the winter, the only means of transport would be dogsled. The people of Nome did have a telegraph so he would need to rely on messages sent by telegraph.[35]

Once Welch became sure the disease he was seeing was diphtheria, he conferred with his nurses, notified the mayor, and made recommendations to establish a temporary board of health. The board acted on Welch's recommendations to implement measures such as closing public buildings, minimizing public gatherings, discouraging movement along trails by children, and limiting adult movement to only official business. The nurses tracked down suspicious cases and reported them to the board of health. All houses with cases were placarded, and quarantine was instituted. Any patient with inflammation of the throat was provisionally quarantined.[36]

As the Strangling Angel's march into Nome continued, the people turned to the sled dog teams of Alaska to fight the challenges of terrain, time, and disease to get the vitally needed serum to the people of Nome to prevent an epidemic. The survival of the men and their dogs, as well as the children of Nome, would depend on the human-animal partnership.

The Mushers and the Dogs

Alaskan mushers and their dogs had opened the Alaska frontier.[37] Just as in the Old West the horse meant freedom for the American cowboy, the sled dog meant freedom and independence to Alaskans.[38] The relationship between a musher and his sled dog was one of mutual respect. The musher respected the dog as a dog. The sled dog provided for mushers' livelihood, helped transport food and supplies, and occasionally carried a sick person to care. Some dogs assisted in hauling freight outside the mining camps.

The ability of the dogs to work well as a team created their power and the lead dog created the team. A good lead dog set the pace, built team confidence, and was smart. A lead dog worked for the master and for the good of the team. The role required courage and was not suitable for a timid or tentative dog. The lead dog needed to be strong-willed, bold, and able to concentrate on the task.

Even smaller dogs could be a lead dog if they were bold enough. It was the spirit of the dog that made the difference. The lead dog developed a special relationship with the musher and set the tone for the team.[39] Lead dogs and their mushers became Alaska's sports heroes.

Seppala

Dogsledding was the favorite entertainment in Alaska in 1925, and Leonhard Seppala was its rock star. Seppala was the head trainer and owner of dogs at the Hammer Consolidated Mining Company. Because of his sled dog racing success, Seppala was a legendary sled dog musher in Alaska.[40] He was often photographed in his parka with his dogs beside him.

Seppala was born in Norway in 1877 and grew up self-reliant and tough, helping his blacksmith father with farm work. His father also earned a living as a fisherman and was gone for extended periods. The call of the gold rush reached young Seppala, and he arrived in Alaska to search for gold in 1900. He began working for the Pioneer Mining Company and learned to mine. Seppala drove dogs between the mining camps, moving supplies and transporting miners who needed medical attention to Nome.[41] It was rugged and physical work. Seppala was not a big man—5 foot, 7 inches and about 140 pounds—but he grew strong in his career as a miner. During the gold rush, he had learned to wrestle in self-defense. With light brown wavy hair, he looked weathered but younger than his years. His small appearance was deceiving; he proved to be more than a match for whatever Alaska had to offer.

Seppala became known as a man of courage and enthusiasm with a mischievous twinkle. He smiled often. He had been known to walk down Front Street on his hands and do somersaults to make the kids laugh. Leonhard Seppala loved and respected his dog team. He watched and learned from dogs. His dogs were important to him.[42]

The sport of dogsled racing developed while Seppala was in Alaska. After the excitement of the gold rush was over, Alaska searched for entertainment and recreation. Interest in dog racing increased, and the reputation of racing dogs and men spread over Alaska. The All-Alaska sweepstakes was a course from Nome to the Seward Peninsula and back; it took stamina and speed. Champions and celebrities of the sport were soon born.

Seppala's employer had placed him in charge of the mining company's kennels, raising and training a group of about 15 female Siberian Huskies and puppies. Seppala entered the 1914 Nome sweepstakes and won the second year he tried. It was said that Seppala had hypnotic powers of control over the dogs.[43] He was known as "the king of the Alaskan trail." One year he traveled 7,000 miles of trail on a dogsled. Those who lost races to Seppala's lean, smaller-framed dogs often called them "Seppala's Siberian rats." After one race, Seppala reported hearing one of the other drivers complaining, "He just sat in his sled smoking a cigar while his dogs walked away from us as fresh as though they had just started."[44] Still, those who knew him described him as unassuming and modest, even when fame came both in the United States and abroad.[45]

In the winter of 1925, Nome turned to Seppala, his dogs Togo and Balto, and Alaska's sled dogs and mushers to deliver diphtheria serum and precious hope.

Togo

Of all his dogs, it was Togo who had Seppala's heart. Togo was Seppala's "bad boy made good," an unruly pup who knew how to chase trouble and find it. He was born in Little Creek, Alaska, and was the offspring of Seppala's former lead dog, Suggen. He had been named after a Japanese admiral. Captain Roald Amundsen had planned to make an expedition to the North Pole, and the dog team had been intended to be given to Amundsen to make the voyage. However, when the war came, Amundsen's project and the expedition were canceled, and the dogs were given to Seppala.

Togo was born and raised in Seppala's kennels. From the beginning, Togo was hard to handle. At seven months, Togo still could not focus or obey well enough to make a good sled dog and already had a rowdy reputation.[46]

Although Togo had been bred to be a dogsled dog, that career path was not looking good for the rebellious youngster. Seppala decided that the unruly husky would never make a good sled dog and decided to give Togo away to a woman friend of his to be her companion pet. Togo's career as a lady's pampered house dog would turn out to be brief but eventful.

Although treated to steak dinners, Togo expressed his appreciation to his new mistress by nipping her and successfully executing his escape. Togo missed the open space and ability to roam freely. He broke out through a window and hauled back to Little Creek Mining Kennels to be with Seppala, for whom Togo had developed a fierce loyalty. Seppala had to admit he admired the feisty pup: the young dog was loyal and bold. Seppala had missed him. He allowed Togo to stay.[47] Togo had run and won his first race.

Togo grew up under Seppala's care. The young husky would follow Seppala's team out on their runs, nipping at the dogs' ears to harass them, and then run off to avoid punishment from dog or human. He was clever and fast. He respected Seppala and wanted the boss's attention. If they met a strange team on the trail, Togo would jump at the other lead dog to make way for his beloved Seppala. On one trip, Togo met his match in a team of malamutes, and his behavior got him bit up so severely he had to be carried home in the sled. Seppala recalled, "Togo hated the indignity of having to ride on anything."[48] Togo had learned his lesson, which was an important one for a sled dog leader: the leader has to approach, meet, and pass another team. For the rest of his lead dog career, passing a team going in the same direction, Togo would always get his own team out of the way of the other team, which gave his team the advantage of not allowing another team to catch them.[49]

When Togo was eight months old, Seppala had to go away on a 160-mile business trip of a few days and did not trust the canine delinquent to be around the kennels unsupervised. Seppala asked an assistant to lock Togo in a dog corral while he was away, hoping to prevent any shenanigans. The dog corral had a seven-foot fence with a wire mesh, and Seppala was sure that would hold that pup tight. He told his assistant not to let Togo out.[50]

Togo executed his escape as soon as Seppala left—or tried to. The young dog cleared the tall fence, but his leg was caught in the wire mesh. Squeaking and squirming, Togo complained loudly enough that Seppala's assistant investigated and found the yelping husky hanging on the fence outside the corral. Unrepentant, when he was cut down, Togo rolled over and promptly ran off into the cold arctic night.

Seppala changed tactics. He began letting Togo run with the team. Togo returned the favor by leading the team after a reindeer over a crusty section of trail where even a musher could not stand. When the reindeer was gone and Seppala got himself and the rest of the team untangled, he grabbed an extra harness so he could put the annoying rascal of a dog in a position where he could control him. Seppala finally decided that there was nothing to do but try out the little husky. Again, Seppala put the squirming and rolling Togo in harness. They had gone only a few miles when Seppala promoted him to the lead; by the time they arrived at the destination, Togo led while Rusty, the usual leader, watched. Seppala saw a transformation.

Once in place, Togo ran as if he had been waiting for the chance and had done it all his young life. Seppala observed that the eight-month-old unruly husky focused his brown eyes straight ahead and worked harder than any other member of the team. Seppala was struck by the realization that Togo had been trying to show him something all along. Togo was a born leader.[51]

Togo had earned his place as lead dog.[52] He would bark, yelp, and run ahead and his team understood. Togo could find the trail and sense danger. Togo would become as legendary as Seppala in Alaska and a living legend.[53]

He weighed 48 pounds, small for a Siberian husky and small for a lead dog. He was black-brown and grayish, almost foxlike with a pointed nose and a bushy tail that curled over his back. Togo had an uncanny sense of direction and unquestioned loyalty to Seppala. Seppala trusted Togo so much that Seppala could go to sleep in the sled and Togo would take him safely to their destination. However, if it was a winding trail, one of Togo's strengths became a liability: he would try to eliminate the bends in the path even if it meant climbing an almost vertical bank.[54] Seppala became thankful for one of Togo's faults: the dog had an uncanny ability to find the shortest distance between two points.[55] Togo would lead his team 170 miles east to the rally point and then back along a 91-mile stretch over the most treacherous terrain.

Togo became the most traveled dog in Alaska. By 1925, Togo had been Seppala's lead dog for seven years, was at the height of condition and vigor, and had traveled over most terrain in Alaska.[56] Seppala said that when he rode with Togo, he raced with a sense of security and that the little gray Siberian proved to be his most exceptional leader.

Kenneth Ungermann, in his 1963 book *The Race to Nome,* described the special bond of Seppala and Togo when Seppala looked ahead and saw Togo loping forward before him: "He knew those other dogs were not the equal of Togo; he was the finest trail leader the musher had ever known. There would never be a dog that could replace the Siberian Husky in Seppala's heart."[57]

The serum run would be Togo's last long run.[58]

Balto

Unlikely heroes often appear at their moment in history. Balto was just such a hero. Balto was never considered lead dog or breeding material by Seppala. The boxcar-shaped husky was known for his endurance and ability to run while hauling freight. Balto was big, strong, focused, and disciplined. In 1925, at five years old, he was a sturdy dog with a boxy body with white socks and partial white markings on his belly and top of his muzzle. A white sugar-like dusting would progressively cover his muzzle as he aged. Balto had been bred and raised by Seppala, who did not think Balto fit a racing profile or was breeding material. Seppala had tried Balto on his fast team but did not believe the big husky was qualified, so Balto was assigned to a slow-work team.[59] Balto was assigned a role as a freight dog.

It turned out that Balto's strength and discipline were just what was needed and were called into action to complete the final 53-mile leg of the serum run to Nome. When the decision was made to speed up the rally by adding more teams, Seppala's young assistant, Gunnar Kaasen, chose Balto to lead his team.[60] The serum run was to be held in at least –30-degree weather, and Kaasen thought about what would be important in the coming storm.[61] It was the first time Balto had led a team. He was "just a freighting dog," and the serum run was his first lead-dog assignment.

As the Strangling Angel began its march into Nome, Seppala, Togo, and the unlikely Balto were about to become public health pioneers. Togo and Balto with Seppala and Dr. Welch and his staff would all have a part in protecting the public health of the residents of Nome and health care practice in Alaska. Each of these remarkable individuals had a role to play, but it was the dogs that played pivotal roles in inspiring the public and raising awareness of preventive health to Alaska in the icy winter of 1925.

The Race

On January 22, 1925, Dr. Curtis Welch sent a telegram to the U.S. Public Health Service in Washington, D.C., requesting an emergency supply of anti-serum:

An epidemic of diphtheria is almost inevitable here STOP I am in need of one million units of diphtheria antitoxin STOP Mail is the only form of transportation STOP I have made application to the commissioner of health of the territories for antitoxin already STOP There are about 3000 white natives in the district STOP.[62]

While Nome waited for delivery of the antitoxin, Curtis Welch and his small staff of health care providers battled the diphtheria onslaught. It fell to Morgan and Welch to administer the serum on hand to the community, and it would be Morgan and the small staff who would inoculate Nome once the serum arrived. The epidemic already counted 22 confirmed cases, 20 suspected cases, and five deaths.[63]

The manufacturer of the antitoxin was able to locate a million units of the antitoxin, but the supply was spread out over the Pacific Coast and would never reach Nome in time. Dr. John Bradley Beeson, a surgeon for the Alaska Railroad Hospital in Anchorage, located a supply of 300,000 units of serum in a back room of a storehouse. Wrapped in glass vials, blanketed in quilts, they fit into a metallic cylinder weighing just over 20 pounds.[64]

The dilemma now was how to get the serum to Nome in time. In the winter, Nome could not be reached by sea or air. The only planes were open cockpit and could not be flown. The Alaska railroad offered access only as far as Nenana, a railhead town 674 miles from Nome. The last resort was the Alaska mail route, known as the Iditarod Trail. The only way to travel that trail was by sled dogs and men strong and brave enough to guide them.[65] Thus, the only way to reach Nome was over land: from Seward by train 433 miles north through Alaska to the Athabaskan village of Nenana north of Fairbanks and then by dogsled 674 miles west to Nome.[66]

The governor of Alaska, the mayor of Nome, and other officials debated how to deliver the serum in time. Discarding the idea of air or rail for the entire trip, Governor Scott Cardelle Bone, based on a suggestion from Welch and Nome Mayor George Maynard, decided to use a relay of dogs to handle the overland run. The dogsled run would begin when the train arrived in Nenana. The record for mail delivery on this route was nine days; the usual was 30.

While the small, determined medical team in Nome began inoculating residents against the disease, a team of dogs and mushers was about to respond to its call to destiny. The dogsled relay teams were organized for the run for serum.

Alaska Governor Bone and Nome Mayor Maynard knew Nome needed the best dogs and drivers on earth. High winds could cause whiteouts along the route, and the temperature could drop to deadly levels. Bone and Maynard chose Leonhard Seppala and additional well-known mushers to make up the 20 teams. Seppala was assigned to drive east 170 miles from Nome to get the serum and then go directly back 91 miles.

Seppala chose Togo, his fastest, smartest, and boldest, to lead the most critical and challenging leg of the run with him. Togo led the team 170 miles to the touch point. Preparing for his 91-mile leg on the most treacherous part of the journey, Seppala faced a tough decision. He had to decide whether to take a shortcut over the frozen Norton Sound or to go around the more dangerous route. Gale force winds confronted him, and the ice threatened to break up at any moment.

Seppala was confident in his lead dog. Togo had an exceptional ability to find the trail and an uncanny ability to detect danger. Togo led them across the jagged ice to the safety of land, traveling through blinding snow and gale force wind. Just three hours after they passed, the ice broke on Norton Sound. Seppala handed off the serum to the next relay, who then handed it to Gunnar Kaasen's team.

Kaasen chose Balto to lead his team, knowing that Balto was big, strong, reliable, and had endurance. Seppala disagreed with Kaasen's pick; he did not think Balto was a good enough lead dog. But Balto proved himself. Used to pulling heavy freight, he moved steadfastly through the raging blizzard. At one point he halted and would not go further on a patch of ice. The ice he would not go across later broke. Balto had saved his driver and team from an icy death in the Topkok River. No one expected that Balto and Kaasen would make the leg of the trip through the roaring blizzard so quickly, so when Balto and the team arrived at the safety shelter, they found the next driver asleep. As the team forged on, a fierce blast of arctic wind blasted the sled dogs and sled into the air, and Kaasen almost lost the precious serum in the snow. It had disappeared, but he searched and found it. Exhausted and nearly frozen, Balto led Kaasen's team into Nome just before dawn on February 2, 1925.[67]

The world had watched. News of Nome's problem and the serum run to solve it had been flashed across the United States, and newspaper headlines had reported the team's progress. At its conclusion, 20 mushers and 150 dogs had traveled 674 miles in 5 days and 7½ hours. Many mushers considered it a world record.[68] Balto was the dog the media saw come over the finish line at the end of the run to deliver the serum, and he became a media celebrity.

Once the serum arrived in Nome, it still had to reach the patients. Emily Morgan and the nurses risked their own lives to reach remote villages and communities, entering quarantine zones, calming suspicious families, and administering the doses. Morgan donned layers of woolen clothes, a fur parka, and mucklucks and walked in sub-zero weather to inoculate the residents of Nome. Her nurse's bag contained a flashlight, syringes, tongue depressors, antitoxin, and candy to tempt children. She prayed with some families and helped one father build a coffin for his child. After a miner broke quarantine and sneaked into the red light district, she brought doses to Nome's prostitutes.[69]

Five children were reported to have died, and 29 cases of diphtheria had been diagnosed. One source claimed 11,000 people had been threatened. The serum run was an example of human-animal collaboration under the most brutal conditions toward a humanitarian goal. Trust and communication between human and dog and the leadership of the lead dog had prevented a disaster. Each of the 20 drivers received a medal from the manufacturer of the serum and was honored with a certificate of thanks from President Calvin Coolidge. However, the real reward was that children were playing in Nome again.[70] Balto and Kaasen became instant media celebrities.

The Rest of the Journey

In 1926, Balto and Kaasen made a movie and went on tour in the lower United States. A statue of Balto was erected in Central Park. Eventually, Balto and six other dogs on the team were sold and became the feature in a vaudeville-type sideshow until Cleveland businessman George Kimble, fearing that they were neglected and mistreated, decided to bring them to Cleveland. Kimble needed to raise $2,000 to purchase the team, and a Balto Fund was established. The community rallied around Balto and donations came in from across the country. Children in Cleveland collected coins in buckets. The Western Reserve Kennel Club donated enough to meet a fundraising goal in just 10 days. With the money raised from the campaign, Balto and the other dogs were purchased, brought to Cleveland, and given a hero's welcome with a parade through downtown Cleveland. They lived out their lives at the Brookside Children's Zoo. Balto died in March 1933 at age 14. His body was stuffed and is now at the Cleveland Museum of National History, which produces a brochure, "A Race for Life," about Balto and the serum run.[71]

The serum run had also generated controversy and jealousy among some participants. Mushers had different views about who deserved credit for the achievements. In some cases, the details of the race were related in different versions and were said to have been exaggerated or embellished as various media rushed to report the events as they occurred.[72] Seppala was particularly bitter about the fact that Balto had received the notoriety while Togo had run the longest and hardest leg of the run. The final insult for Seppala was when Balto, not Togo, was pushed into the limelight and immortalized in the bronze statue in New York's Central Park.[73] Balto, not Togo, became a symbol of all the dogs and men and the indomitable spirit that carried the serum 674 miles. Seppala felt that Togo was the real hero dog and wrote that he was both amazed and amused that it was Balto who received the credit. He referred to Balto as a "newspaper dog."[74] The story of Balto has been told in several children's books, and an animated film titled *Balto* is loosely based on Balto. In

2013, a documentary, *Icebound—The Greatest Dog Story Ever Told*, focused on the aftermath of the events.

Seppala decided that Togo should retire and brought the dog to live with Elizabeth Ricker, his kennel partner, friend, and fellow musher in Maine so Togo could enjoy some pampering. Seppala stated that the serum run was Togo's last long run and that he had worked his hardest and his best. Seppala reflected on his parting with Togo:

> It seemed best to leave him where he could be pensioned and enjoy a well-earned rest. But it was a sad parting on a cold gray March morning when Togo raised a small paw to my knee as if questioning why he was not going along with me. For the first time in twelve years, I hit the trail without Togo.[75]

Seppala and his team toured the lower 48 states together, and he continued to race with a team of 44 dogs. He started Seppala Kennels in Poland Spring, Maine, with Elizabeth Ricker and established a Siberian kennel at Poland Spring, which would become the origin of the spread of the Siberian husky breed in the United States and Canada. Harry W. Wheeler's 1931 acquisition of three Siberian huskies together with other breeding stock from Poland Spring became the foundation of the Seppala Strain that was first registered by the Canadian Kennel Club in 1939 as the Siberian husky. Although Seppala's direct involvement with the breed that now bears his name ended, he played a significant part in the birth of the Seppala Siberian sled dog breed in the 1990s.[76]

When sled dog racing became a demonstration event at the Lake Placid Winter Olympics in 1932, Seppala earned a silver medal. After 1932 Seppala remained in Alaska and then moved to Seattle, where he and his wife retired and where he remained until his death in 1967 at the age of 90.[77] He had logged an estimated 250,000 dogsled miles.[78]

On February 16, 1925, Dr. Welch published a letter in the *Journal of the American Medical Association* in which he reported a detailed account of the Nome epidemic and his actions. The letter illustrated the difficulties of medical practice under primitive conditions.[79] Dr. and Mrs. Welch left Nome shortly after the serum run in September 1925 and returned to Alaska in 1927 for two years until, for health reasons, they moved to Santa Barbara, California. They returned to Alaska during summers to relieve vacationing doctors or to visit friends. Dr. Welch continued to be received as a hero in Alaska. After a period of ill health, Dr. Welch died at age 70 in 1948. Lulu Welch moved into a retirement home and lived there until her death in 1958. She sent her memoirs to the Alaska Nurses Association.

After the Nome epidemic subsided, Emily Morgan returned to Kansas to resume her career in Red Cross nursing. Emily Morgan became known as "the Angel of the Yukon" for her work administering the serum to the natives of Alaska. Over the years, she returned to Alaska to care for the sick. She was called back to Nome to help fight a smallpox epidemic in Northern Alaska; she also served as a missionary nurse in New Zealand. She never married and died in 1960 at the age of 82. She was inducted into the Alaska Women's Hall of Fame in 2013.

Legacy: Public Health

The diphtheria epidemic and serum run of 1925 was one of the 20th century's most significant demonstrations of the unique contribution of dogs working with humans in a public health crisis that shaped public health history.[80] The dogs, men, and women of the serum run fought challenges of weather, terrain, disease, and time—and won. It was an example of human-animal cooperation that affected public health.[81]

News of the courage of Togo and Balto and the other team members sparked a national vaccine campaign. Transportation of medical supplies and vaccines is key to health care delivery. It is especially challenging in remote areas during catastrophes or natural or manmade disasters. The challenge of distribution, as well as supply in an emergency, was illustrated in Nome, and the dog teams represented a trusted, community resource that was uniquely available to solve the problem. The serum race also provided impetus to pass the Kelly Act, which was signed into law and allowed private aviation companies in Alaska to bid on mail delivery contracts. The day after the serum run, the Associated Press reported that the post office was implementing plans for airmail service to Alaska.[82] The technology of transportation improved, and air routes were eventually established in Alaska.

In 1955, the responsibility for health service for Alaskan natives was transferred from the Bureau of Indian Affairs Alaska Native Service to the U.S. Public Health Service. The Public Health Service played a significant role in the serum run and in further ramping up public health prevention efforts in Alaska.[83] The 1925 annual report of the Public Health Service emphasized that many lives were lost due to diphtheria, which could be saved by timely access to diphtheria antitoxin. Nurses traveled to villages teaching about good health and providing medical assistance and immunizations. New hospitals were built, and a community health aide program was established. Doctors and nurses began to make regular field trips, and a regular radio medical network was developed.

The publicity from the serum run and the heroic contribution of the dogs prompted a national campaign in the 1930s to use diphtheria vaccine.[84] It became routinely used by the 1940s after being combined with tetanus and pertussis (whooping cough) vaccines.[85] In the end, hundreds of lives in the community in and around Nome were saved because people in Alaska and across the United States worked together.

The events raised awareness of the public health infrastructure for rural health care outreach and supply distribution and communication. Until 1925, there were 210,000 cases of diphtheria with 20,000 deaths annually in the United States.[86] The serum run galvanized the people in the United States to begin using the diphtheria vaccine, and as a result, diphtheria has been virtually wiped out in the country.[87]

Today, the U.S. Centers for Disease Control and Prevention still features the story of the "Great Race of Mercy," which "celebrates the achievement of the dogs and men in public health history."[88] Today the Alaska "Race to Vaccinate" campaign raises awareness of the need for timely vaccination for children before the age of 2 years old. The "I Did It by TWO!" immunization campaign features the serum race in its campaign to vaccinate children by age 2 as part of a cooperative education effort of the Alaska Immunization Program, the Alaska Nurses Association, and the Vaccinate Alaska Coalition.[89]

It fell to the dogs, men, nurses, and people of Alaska to demonstrate the teamwork, leadership, and courage required to save Nome. The message brought to life by the dogsled run was clear: transportation, communication, and collaboration are critical to the health of Alaska and to other rural and frontier areas. The courage, intelligence, and fortitude of the sled dogs as public servants, each with their own unique strengths, blended into a team that left an enduring health care legacy across the wilderness of Alaska in 1925. They transformed public health in Alaska with their contribution to mass immunization public health education and awareness and affected the history of vaccinology.[90]

In health care, few real improvements are accomplished without leadership, teamwork, and determination. Togo and Balto and their partnership with men showed us what leadership and cooperation look like. They showed Americans what they needed to do—and how to get there. As public servants, they provided a model of leadership training, loyalty, and safety that underpins all successful health care.

Since 1973, the Iditarod Trail race has run annually and is a memorial to the sled dogs and mushers of 1925. Although it does not follow the same path as the serum run, the Iditarod commemorates the serum run.[91] The dogs used in the Iditarod today are known as Alaskan huskies. They're small, short-haired dogs, seldom weighing more than 50 pounds. Their best-known traits are a blend of speed and endurance, tough feet, and an almost unbelievable ability to withstand cold.[92]

There may be more to learn from mushers and their dogs. In a 2011 study, Kuhl investigated the elements and quality of musher and sled dog relationships.[93] Eight mushers were asked to contribute by sharing their stories and experiences working with sled dogs. The researcher found that there are unique elements in human–working dog relationships and that these relationships can have many nuances that are rich and deep in quality. The study also found that interspecies relationships are significant.

The researcher concluded that building relationships between humans and other animals is vital because of the implications for how humans see and perceive both other animals and fellow humans. While all research subjects had their own perspectives, six themes emerged about the mushers' relationships with their dogs: (1) the importance of getting to know the dogs, (2) respect for sled dogs' abilities, (3) the need for two-way communication, (4) the importance of trust, (5) the notion of partnership, and (6) learning from working with sled dogs.

Critical issues and questions surround the mutuality of the human-animal bond and the humane treatment of animals in human work and entertainment. Opportunities exist today for open discussion and exploration of the humane issues surrounding dogs who work with and for humans. In recent years, the debate has opened up on the humane implications of the treatment of dogs in the Iditarod race and dogsledding. Critics and advocates differ on whether the sport demonstrates humane treatment of the dogs. Open dialogue and examination of humane issues involved in our partnership with working dogs can improve our interspecies collaboration with dogs as sentient beings, not objects. As humans continue to study and discuss how best to care for and protect our canine partners, we may learn more about what we owe them in return for their devotion, courage, and service.

A sled dog team and a health care team have a great deal in common. Both must be high performing and demand influential leaders who can show the way through difficult terrain and rapidly respond to a crisis in the right direction. Both rely on teamwork, safety, communication, training, efficiency, and finding the proper role for each team member's talent.

Togo, Balto, and the teams were symbols and teachers for collaboration and teamwork. When Togo and Balto and their human and canine teammates showed Alaska the way out of the darkness of a diphtheria epidemic, they became a metaphor for the enduring and indomitable spirit of Alaska. They inspired a country and the world when hope was elusive when days were dark, and when the children of Nome were isolated with no apparent way to reach them. Hearing the call, they overcame the challenge of terrain, time, and temperature. They each found the role they were destined to play. They improved critical transportation infrastructure, and they raised awareness of immunization and public health.

The sled dogs of Alaska also showed the power of a hero's journey. Each hero heard his own call. Watching the mushers and sled dogs of the serum run showed us about interspecies communication, teamwork, courage, leadership, endurance, and loyalty. Future teams of humans and working dogs

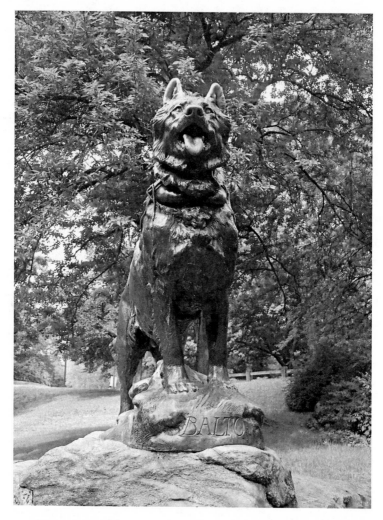

On December 17, 1925, Balto was present when this statue by Frederick Roth was dedicated in Central Park in New York City where it still stands today (© Uris [English Wikipedia]).

may one day reveal more opportunities for human-dog collaboration and the power of the interspecies connection to health care.

The glowing bronze statue of Balto erected in 1925 to commemorate the dogs and mushers of the serum run still stands in Central Park in New York City.

5

Buddy: The Guide Dog
Who Pioneered a New Frontier

Young Morris Frank's cockiness about his dog Buddy got under the reporter's skin. Morris Frank was blind, and he and Buddy had just made a triumphant crossing of the Atlantic from Vevey, Switzerland, and Buddy arrived as the first Seeing Eye dog in America. Frank had trained with Buddy for five weeks in Switzerland and was ready to begin work to establish a Seeing Eye dog program in the United States. Buddy, a German shepherd dog, had been the hit of the ship during the crossing.

Frank and Buddy returned to America with two objectives: to show that dogs were safe to guide blind people and to get guide dogs accepted in public places. When their ship docked in New York Harbor on June 11, 1928, a crowd of reporters met them. On arrival in New York, the pair encountered skeptics, distractions, and noises that Buddy had never seen or heard. American reporters doubted that any dog, much less a German shepherd, could be trusted to be responsible for a "helpless" blind man.

Morris Frank had granted one interview. The reporter dared Frank to try to cross hazardous West Street. Frank, unaware that the street had no stoplights, had plenty of horse-drawn carriages and exploded with waterfront traffic, was undaunted. "Brother, you show us where it is, and we'll cross it."[1]

Frank and the reporter went to the curb outside the dock. Frank commanded Buddy, "Forward." The pair hit a barrage of roaring motors, horse hooves, screeching tires, rims against cobblestones, and shouts from motorists.[2] Buddy backed up hard and pulled Frank away from a truck. She then moved on, her head moving side to side. Frank could feel her actions through her harness. Buddy watched for the danger and led Frank ahead. By this time, Frank had lost all sense of direction, but he knew he could count on his guide dog. They negotiated the trip across to the corner and to a waiting taxi. Frank later said those few moments were the longest of his life. "I lost all sense of direction and surrendered myself entirely to the dog."[3]

Frank had a good reason for his confidence in his dog. On their trans-Atlantic journey, Buddy had already shown Frank that a blind man could count on a trained guide dog to find his way in the world. While still on board the ship, Frank cashed a check at the purser and then returned to his cabin for a nap. As Frank stretched out on his berth, Buddy touched him with her paw. At first, Frank ignored her. Then she reached up with her paws and dropped something onto his chest. It was his wallet. He had dropped it on the floor in the purser's office, and no one but Buddy had noticed. Buddy had acted on her own initiative and traveled the length of the deck to bring it back to him.[4]

From New York, Buddy and Frank made their way home to Nashville. On the way back home, they stopped in multiple cities to introduce Buddy to the world. They returned to their Nashville home as conquering heroes, having traveled thousands of miles using all kinds of transportation. Buddy had demonstrated that a well-educated guide dog could guide a blind person safely through some of the biggest and most complicated cities in the world.

Morris Frank knew where he was going and his dog was going with him to lead the way. He said he had "signed my declaration of independence" and planned to enjoy life to the fullest.[5] *His quest to establish a guide dog school for the blind in the United States had begun.*[6] *Those who lacked sight did not need to be helpless. Buddy would show America how it was done.*[7] *Buddy, the first Seeing Eye dog in the United States, and Morris Frank were about to demonstrate a human-animal bond that served to help thousands of blind people achieve independence. What Buddy and Frank would accomplish would soon set a standard for the world to follow.*

When they had arrived home, the next morning Buddy and Frank rose early and hopped a streetcar bound for Western Union. They met the clerk at the desk, and Frank told him,

"I want to send a cable."

"Yes, sir, what's the message?"

"SUCCESS."

"Is that all, just one word?"

"Brother, that tells everything."[8]

Beginnings

The journey to establish the first Seeing Eye dog school in America began with a trio of unlikely pioneers. The partners were a young blind man who yearned for the freedom to live his life independently, a petite, genteel, charming well-to-do woman on a Swiss mountain thousands of miles away, a snuff-chewing trainer who had once been a cowboy, and a female German shepherd dog named Buddy who was once called Kiss. Together with Dorothy

Eustis as president and Jack Humphrey as vice president of training and research, Morris Frank with Buddy at his side founded The Seeing Eye, the first guide dog school in the United States. Today, The Seeing Eye, Inc. remains the oldest existing guide dog school in the world.[9]

Frank and Buddy demonstrated that the consequences of enhanced and safe mobility were dignity, self-confidence, and independence. They also worked to shape public policy on granting public accommodation to those who use the service of a guide dog.[10]

The trio's paths first intersected on a night in 1927. On November 15, Morris Frank's father sat in the living room of the Frank house on Richland Avenue in Nashville and began to read the *Saturday Evening Post* to his blind son. Frank's father read, stopping twice to compose himself and to clear his voice that had grown husky: "This is called 'The Seeing Eye.'" He read aloud Dorothy Harrison Eustis's article[11] describing how the Germans had trained shepherd dogs to take the place of a blind person's eyes. Eustis was a breeder and trainer of German shepherd dogs in Switzerland.

Morris Frank sat transfixed in his living room. His entire attention focused on absorbing the words his father read. He listened to Eustis's description of harnesses with a curved leather handle that became a link between a dog and his or her blind master—a lifeline to the blind. As he heard his father read, Morris Frank saw freedom, and he saw a dog—and his dream of a dog lit up his darkness.

The young blind man heard a life-altering message that night. He heard hope and a new life. He could hardly believe it. It must be a miracle that these dogs could lead the master by detecting hazards and preventing their master from moving if it was not safe. He imagined a dog taking the place of a human attendant. Obtaining such a dog could mean the end of the humiliation of continual dependence on others. It could mean a new life of freedom for a young man who dreamed of independence.

Morris Frank could not see, but he had a vision. He saw a different future for himself. He could dream. He dreamed of being able to date a girl and kiss her goodnight at her door without a guard to crowd his space. Frank had to have an escort when he dated a girl. This meant he could not be alone with her. Looking at this escort while kissing his date goodnight at the end of an evening that had been accompanied by an escort was not the social life Frank envisioned. He wanted to deliver his date to her front door and return to his car like a man. He wanted self-respect.

Morris Frank

Frank was born in Tennessee and was the youngest son of wealthy parents. When he was 6 years old, he lost vision in one eye in a horseback riding accident and lost the sight in his second eye in a boxing match when he was 16. Frank's mother was also blind from the time Frank was 3 years old. Frank attended Vanderbilt University in Nashville and sold insurance door to door while he was a student. Now, as a young man in his 20s, he yearned to break out of the prison of blindness, and he thought others in America would want that too. Morris dreamed of attending his college classes without a paid attendant to go with him, to visit clients without a talkative escort. He dreamed of being able to go where he wanted. He dreamed of being seen as himself, not just a blind person. A dog like that described by Dorothy Eustis could open frontiers he thought were forever closed to him.

Frank's father paused his reading of the *Saturday Evening Post* article. Morris's mother joined them in the living room and sat beside him without saying a word. Frank's mother understood what life as a blind person meant and what freedom could mean to a blind person. Morris's mother had also been blinded accidentally, having lost her first eye when a blood vessel burst during the birth of a child and losing the second in a fall from a horse.

The three Franks just looked at each other. They understood what such a dog could mean to all of them. Frank's father's voice broke just one more time as he finished reading. Everyone in the room sat in silence for several minutes. Then they all began to talk at once.

Frank was determined to get such a dog.[12] He was planning to change his life, and he needed a dog to be his partner. That night, instead of sleeping, Frank tossed and turned all night.[13] The next morning Morris's father typed as Morris dictated a letter to Mrs. Eustis in care of *The Saturday Evening Post*.

> Is what you say really true? If so, I want one of those dogs! Also, I am not alone. Thousands of blind like me abhor being dependent on others. Help me, and I will help them. Train me, and I will bring back my dog and show people here how a blind man can be entirely on his own. We can then set up an instruction center in this country to give all those here who want it a chance at a new life.[14]

Frank's hand shook as he signed his name to the most important letter of his life. He tapped his way with his cane to the mailbox in his neighborhood. He dropped the letter and his hopes into the mailbox and spent the next 30 long days waiting for a reply.

Finally, Mrs. Eustis replied that she had never trained dogs for the blind, but that if Frank dared to come all the way from Tennessee to Switzerland in search of a dog, she had a qualified trainer to work with him. When Eustis telephoned two weeks later to talk with Frank, she said with a quiet voice, "Mr. Frank, do you still think you want to come to Switzerland for your dog? It's a very long trip for a blind boy alone." Frank almost shouted into the phone, "Mrs. Eustis, to get back my independence, I'd go to hell."[15]

Blind in America

Morris Frank, blind and alone, sailed for Switzerland in April 1928, accepting Eustis's invitation to visit her school and begin his quest for a guide dog for himself. Morris Frank was a frustrated and angry traveler. He was classified on the ship's manifest as a parcel.

As Morris Frank began his trans-Atlantic voyage, blind people were considered helpless and not capable of functioning independently. A ship steward was assigned to supervise Morris Frank's every move. Frank described the steward as less of an attendant and more of a jailer[16]—the steward would not let the young man do any activity unaccompanied and would exercise the blind young man as if he were a horse, methodically trotting him about the ship deck for exercise. Frank was a young man with a young man's pursuits, and a constant attendant did not help. When Frank met an English girl with whom he wanted to be alone, he could not escape his jailer.[17]

Blindness can have many causes. Some people lose their sight through accidents or war injuries; others, through diseases. Not all kinds of blindness are suitable for the help of a Seeing Eye dog. The decision must be determined case by case. It is possible to be legally blind and still see colors, perceive light, or recognize faces. The most common forms of blindness that affect Seeing Eye graduates are retinopathy of prematurity, retinitis pigmentosa, glaucoma, retinal detachment, and diabetes.[18]

Blind people were marginalized in America in 1923.[19] Institutes for the education of blind children, such as the Perkins School in New Orleans, were established by 1924, but they isolated blind children. Many schools were still called asylums. The Perkins School had been chartered by the Massachusetts legislature in 1829.[20] It had been founded as the New England Asylum for the Blind.[21]

Morris Frank taught himself how to use a white cane for travel. Although the use of the white cane was introduced in France after World War I, it had still been unknown in America. The first city ordinance to grant users of a white cane the right of way was passed in Peoria, Illinois, in 1930. Louis Braille invented the code given his name in 1829, but books for blind persons were coded in five different alphabets until 1917 when an international conference agreed on a single Braille system. Talking books did not exist. The American Federation for the Blind was a young organization, and there were no Braille watches.

Agencies for the blind often regarded their clients as "helpless or afflicted." The phrase "the blind" implied a handicap so terrible it wiped out all individual distinctions to those it "afflicted," who were not seen as individuals.

Morris Frank did not share this philosophy. He did not consider himself "just one of the blind." He was offered a job selling brooms, but he decided

to sell insurance instead. He attended Vanderbilt University. He taught himself Braille.[22] Morris Frank yearned for an independent life. He saw his future,
and it included independence and a guide dog, like one that Dorothy Eustis
had described in her article.

The indignity Morris Frank suffered on his ship journey made him more
determined to establish his independence. However, he realized he could not
do it alone. He was determined to cross the Atlantic alone in search of just
the right partner. This awkward ship crossing would be the last journey Frank
would make without the canine who was about to change his life.[23]

Dorothy Eustis, Jack Humphrey and Fortunate Fields

Dorothy Eustis was breeding and training working German shepherd
dogs at Fortunate Fields when she wrote the article about guide dogs for the
blind for *The Saturday Evening Post,* which caught Morris Frank's attention.
Using dogs to assist the blind was not new. A guide dog is "a domestic dog
which is educated to provide mobility support to a person who is blind or
visually impaired."[24] While some attempts to train dogs to assist blind people
occurred in France and Vienna, the modern guide dog story started in World
War I with the German effort to train dogs to help blind soldiers who had
returned from the front.

Gerhard Stalling, a German doctor, is credited with pioneering the modern guide dog movement. He developed a way to train dogs to work with soldiers to help them become more mobile and live lives after the war. Dr.
Stalling's dog first showed him the way. Stalling was walking a patient on
hospital grounds one day and was called away, but left his dog with the blind
patient as company. Stalling returned and saw that the dog had been looking
after the blind person. Stalling got the idea to train dogs to help blind soldiers
and started training dogs to become reliable guides.[25] He opened the first
guide dog school in Oldenburg, Germany, in 1916.[26] The school expanded in
several locations to provide dogs to blind people all over the world. Another
successful large dog school had opened in Potsdam. The intelligence and
usefulness of the German shepherd dog caught the attention of the public in
the work the Germans were doing with blind soldiers. German shepherd
dogs had herded sheep in Central Europe for two centuries. They were also
used to guard farms and homes, herd, kill rats, and track fugitives.[27]

Dorothy Eustis had already begun training dogs for the military and
police and customs service in Switzerland when she heard about the Potsdam
experience. She was curious about the methods and spent several months
there observing their techniques.

Dorothy Harrison Eustis was petite, wealthy, refined, friendly, and formidable. She spoke with a low voice, but when she did speak, Eustis was direct and clear. The youngest of six children, she was raised in a prominent old Philadelphia family; she married at age 20 and was widowed at age 29. Eight years later, she married George Eustis. In 1923, she and her family moved to a small village called Mount Pelerin, which overlooked Vevey, Switzerland. In 1923, she acquired a beloved purebred German shepherd named Hans who lived to the age of 14. He became the inspiration for her love of the German shepherd breed and one of her first teachers. As she began to observe Hans, Eustis became interested in breeding and established a breeding and training program for German shepherds. She named it Fortunate Fields.[28]

As part of her breeding program, Eustis conducted research. She was interested in breeding and training German shepherds as working dogs rather than show dogs. She learned about what the Germans were doing training guide dogs for the blind as teammates. She had research and interest but needed help. Eustis realized that to take her program where she wanted to go, she needed a trainer.

She found the man she was looking for in Jack Humphrey. Eustis hired experienced American trainer and geneticist Humphrey to develop their scientific approach to breeding and training working German shepherd dogs. Jack Humphrey became the first Seeing Eye trainer and geneticist and chief instructor. Humphrey and Eustis further refined Stalling's approach and introduced the guide dog concept around the world.[29]

Humphrey's background was as colorful and rugged as Dorothy Eustis's was genteel and refined. He usually had snuff behind his upper lip, which earned him the nickname "the cowboy with the weeping lip." He had gray-blue eyes, his ears stuck out, he was just below medium height, and he had the bowlegs of a cowboy. He had an eclectic resume. In Saratoga Springs, he had worked as an apprentice jockey in racing seasons. He went west and broke horses and at one point trained lions for a man who sold animals to the circus. It was said that he had once taught a camel to walk backward. He was an avid reader and compensated for his lack of education by being well read and a keen observer of events around him.[30]

Humphrey was an experienced breeder and trainer. He had bred and trained Arabian horses for a millionaire in New Hampshire. During World War I, he was an army sergeant in charge of animals, and in World War II he was a lieutenant commander in the coast guard serving as an advisor to the canine corps.[31]

Humphrey used a scientific approach to dog breeding. In his 1934 book, *Working Dogs: An Attempt to Produce a Strain of German Shepherds Which Combine Working Ability and Beauty of Conformation*, written with Lucian

Warner, Humphrey published training and breeding methods for working dogs.[32] Humphrey concluded in *Working Dogs* that although dogs are probably more intelligent than any other animal, it is their desire to please that makes them so teachable rather than their intelligence.[33]

In 1924, *Scientific American* published an article, "The German Shepherd Dog," that described breeding programs and the value of the working dog.[34] The publication of Humphrey's findings on training the German shepherd caught the attention of Dorothy Eustis. She read about Humphrey's findings on the genetics of German shepherds and became intrigued by Humphrey's theories on breeding them. After corresponding by letter, Humphrey decided to come in person to see her dogs. The pair eventually agreed on a working partnership, and Humphrey moved with his wife and daughter to Fortunate Fields and began breeding Fortunate Fields German shepherds for working roles.

The first dogs produced at Fortunate Fields were used for military purposes. The program then turned to training dogs to assist the blind. Although by the end of the war the Germans had used 48,000 German shepherd dogs, Fortunate Fields was the first systematic attempt to breed the dogs for work, or for any purpose other than conformation.[35]

The Fortunate Fields partnership worked. The Seeing Eye dog-breeding program had several features that led to success. Although Dorothy Eustis and Jack Humphrey came to Fortunate Fields from different worlds and each possessed a unique style and approach, both were strong-willed, active, analytical, and hard workers. Both were highly interested in breeding good working qualities in German shepherds. They had a shared sense of purpose; they believed in German shepherd dogs and thought their energy was being put to waste when the focus was on beauty rather than utility. They did not plan to sell dogs, so Fortunate Fields could remain independent and not have to breed to any required standard for show dogs.

Humphrey's idea of an ideal dog was different from the standard shepherd bred for the show ring. He felt the large size required for the show ring weakened endurance in the working dog, but he did not allow his theories to blind him if a good dog caught his attention. Humphrey sought and purchased breeding stock of six distinct strains to open up the bloodlines and offer sufficient genetic variety for his working dogs.[36] He did not believe in inline breeding; he thought that the finer qualities of the working dog had been lost through line breeding and inbreeding. He preferred dogs of average size, strong enough to do the dog's work.

Word of the breeding program at Fortunate Fields reached America. In the summer of 1927, the editors of the *Saturday Evening Post* asked Dorothy if she could write a human-interest story on dogs for their publication. She agreed. It would be a turning point in her life.

Although the publisher probably envisioned an article about the breeding work, Dorothy Eustis felt that such an article would have led to requests to buy Fortunate Fields dogs. These dogs were "not for sale and might later be needed for a breeding program."[37] Eustis decided to focus instead on efforts to train dogs for the blind. She had visited the guide dog school at Potsdam, Germany, the school for German military veterans who were blinded during World War I. She wrote how she had been skeptical but completely converted when she saw how a blind person and a German shepherd guide dog could work together to travel a busy and hazardous street. She concluded the article by praising the program and noting the independence it offered to those who were blind:

> The future for all blind men can be the same, however blinded. No longer dependent on a member of the family, a friend or a paid attendant, the blind can once more take up their normal lives as nearly as possible where they left them off, and each can begin or go back to a wage-earning occupation, secure in the knowledge that he can get to and from his work safely and without cost; that crowds and traffic have no longer any terrors for him and that his evenings can be spent among friends without responsibility or burden to them; and last, but far from least, that long, healthful walks are now possible to exercise off the unhealthy fat of inactivity and so keep the body strong and fit. Gentlemen, again without reservation, I give you the shepherd dog.[38]

She chose the title of her article from a Bible verse: "The hearing ear, and the seeing eye, the Lord hath made both of them." Eustis wrote the article, put it in the mail, left for a summer holiday, and forgot about it. She had started a chain of events that led to the introduction of the seeing-eye dog in the United States.

When Eustis's article ran in the *Saturday Evening Post* on November 15, 1927, letters poured in. Bundles of letters deluged Eustis from all over the country, inquiring about getting a Seeing Eye dog. She asked Humphrey, "Jack, what have I done?"[39]

Her attempt to avoid attention had failed. She worried that she had raised the hope of many people who were blind when she was not in a position to help. Or so she thought. The idea of a school for guide dogs in America had been born and was moving fast. Nevertheless, she would be confronted with obstacles, resistance, and skepticism at every turn.

The idea of a dog assisting a blind person would be new to America and not an easy concept to introduce. Using German shepherd dogs to help the blind was an issue in America. The German shepherd breed had an image problem; some associated them with police, guard, or attack dogs. Dorothy tried to interest American agencies in the merits of these dogs but continued to meet resistance. Then she read a letter from a young man in America— Morris Frank. Soon the young man with a dream in search of a dog was on his way across the ocean.

Buddy: The Making of a Guide Dog

Dorothy Eustis and Jack Humphrey knew that the dog that was going to show Americans the value of the German shepherd dog for the blind was going to need intelligence, courage, and character. They had two dogs to choose from, Kiss and Gala. They decided on Kiss, a handsome dark gray German shepherd. Kiss had a busy, graceful tail that swept in an S curve, velvet ears, dark brown eyes, and a creamy patch on her throat.

Morris Frank arrived in the small village outside Vevey, Switzerland. The next morning he had breakfast and set out to meet the dog who would change his life. Eustis and Humphrey told Frank that first, he had to make friends with the dog. He was to pat her and talk to her. He brought raw meat as a friend's offering.

Frank sat in a chair, meat in hand, and heard the sound of soft dog paws on the floor. The door opened and in walked the beautiful dark gray German shepherd. The dog came right to him. A cold nose sniffed his hand and began to eat daintily as he felt the lap of a warm, wet tongue.[40] Morris Frank said,

"What's her name?

"Kiss," Jack Humphrey replied.

"Kiss, that's a hell of a name for a dog."[41]

Frank put his arms around his dog, felt her soft fur, and then said he could not imagine being with his friends and calling "Kiss" every time he wanted his dog so he would name her Buddy. He spent the rest of the day making a fuss over her, and that night she seemed pleased being taken to sleep behind his bed instead of in the dog's quarters. The next morning Frank woke to a warm tongue licking his face.[42]

Buddy and Frank had much to learn. Jack Humphrey believed that the handler must genuinely understand his dog, and the dog needed to be helped to learn what the handler wanted. It would take solid teamwork, time, courage, and patience.

Before training of any guide dog team occurs, puppies must be raised and trained. The foundation of the program was breeding a well-socialized pup that could also focus on the work. When the Fortunate Fields puppies were weaned, they were sent to farm families to raise and grow socialized to life in a family and contact with people. They returned to Fortunate Fields to complete their training. The police, military, or Red Cross dogs were sent onto their assignments once trained and graduated successfully, but Fortunate Fields retained the breeding rights.[43]

The training of the human end of the leash began as students learned to use a white cane. The cane is used by visually handicapped persons to navigate their environment.[44] It is used to check for an object in the person's path, changes in the walking surface, and curbs and steps. A white cane also alerts others that the user of the cane is visually challenged. Along with using the white cane, the student had to learn to command the dog and develop a bond with his or her new partner. Instructors also had to have a bond with the dog.[45]

The harness is a critical component of the communication between handler and dog. The Juno harness is a U-shaped harness that both student and instructor can handle as they walk together in training sessions. A dog in harness continues in a given direction as directed by his handler. The dog also keeps his handler safe from hazards such as manholes.[46] The harness and handle allow a person who cannot see to feel when the dog is stopping, starting, and changing direction. Dogs in the past were on flexible leashes, which meant the dogs could guide in a general direction, but there was no way for dogs to steer their masters away from danger.[47]

A guide dog must learn several commands: forward, right, and left. They practice touch and go—to pause slightly and then continue. The handler must learn to judge traffic movements and sounds. At the right time, the handler commands the dog to go forward. The dog does not read traffic lights. Dogs must stop when the team reaches a stairway so the human can get his footing. The dogs have to stay focused and concentrate and cannot be frightened by loud noises. A blind person and dog must stop and ask for directions just like anyone else. The blind person directs the dog where to go. Rounded curbs present a challenge. If a curb does not have sharp edges or defined corners, the dog can become confused and go in the wrong direction.[48]

Training was strict in Fortunate Fields. The dogs were being prepared to make life-and-death decisions. The instruction at Fortunate Fields was different from other training methods that taught command and obey. A guide dog was trained to "command and obey—if it is okay."[49] This lesson in "intelligent disobedience" was their most important lesson.[50] Dogs had to learn to judge a situation and not obey if the command placed their owner in danger.[51]

Not only did the dogs have to be teachable and receptive to learning, but so did their teachers. Instructors began their day feeding and playing with their canine trainees, and each instructor typically was responsible for 8 to 10 dogs. Even Jack Humphrey learned along the way. Sometimes an instructor would give a small physical nonverbal cue to a dog inadvertently through his body language at the same time he issued a voice command—and the dogs would respond to the physical signal. After that, the team was required to pass a mandatory traffic test with the instructor blindfolded before a dog could graduate.

Dogs found to be unsuitable for guide dog work did not graduate; they became available for adoption. In the early days at Fortunate Fields, they would be given to local farm families. Today, the Seeing Eye considers adoption applications. The average working life of a guide dog is 7 to 8 years,[52] and at the end of his working life he may be given to a friend or today may be returned to the Seeing Eye and rehomed through dog adoption.

Buddy and Frank trained for 6 weeks. Fortunate Fields training was intense since the duo had to be prepared to impress skeptics in America. Buddy and Frank had their share of training mishaps as learners often do, but theirs was a partnership that endured. Frank made mistakes, and Buddy pulled him out of trouble more than once. The first time Buddy and Frank went out on their own, Frank took two steps and ran right into a post. Frank found it took practice to get the harness on and off the patiently waiting Buddy. He poked Buddy in the eye a few times and punched her in the ear.[53]

Eventually Frank increased his handling skill. His concentration and focus improved, and he could tune into Buddy's head movement. Buddy and Frank became familiar faces on the cobblestone streets of the little city as they traveled the itineraries Jack Humphrey laid out for them.

While Jack Humphrey taught that handlers must understand their dog, Frank found out that was not so easy and made several mistakes, witnessed by Humphrey. Frank sat in a cable car next to Buddy on the way home and allowed Buddy to flop down in front of him without making sure that her feet were well out of the way of any passerby. Humphrey stepped on Buddy's paw, and she yelped. Frank then put Buddy under his knees as he was supposed to do and sat there dejected. Humphrey did not speak. Frank was feeling unfairly treated even after returning home. In Morris Frank's memoir, he recalls what Humphrey said:

> Look, you have your choice: you can be just another blind man, or you can be on your own with Buddy's eyes to help you. You cannot lean on me. If I have to follow you and tell you everything, you aren't going to depend on your dog. You won't be able to master the signals. When you go back to the US I won't be there—the future is up to you.[54]

Frank was embarrassed. That night, for the first time he felt discouraged and homesick and wondered if he could ever learn to use a guide dog. Buddy knew. She got up from her place by Frank's bed, crawled in on top of the covers beside him, nuzzled the back of his neck, snuggled as close as she could, and gave a long, low grunt of contentment and companionship. Frank's attitude changed. He realized he had not done so badly, and even Humphrey had admitted he was doing a pretty good job. Buddy had shown him that if he learned his part, they would travel together in safety. He drifted off to sleep with the comfort of Buddy close beside him, support that most dog owners know well. It was the real beginning of the partnership—a man, a dog, and a new world.[55]

Buddy and Morris Frank bonded as they navigated the traffic stairways and crowded streets. They practiced negotiating high curbs and winding streets on the shores of Lake Geneva. One day in training while walking on a narrow road, a runaway horse attached to a cart ran toward them. Buddy pulled Frank up a steep embankment.

When Frank returned to Nashville, his life had changed. He and Buddy negotiated the busy streets and sidewalks with confidence. The formerly helpless man who had needed a paid attendant to accompany him and had traveled across the sea as a parcel had transformed into a confident and independent man.

The world had opened up for Frank and Buddy. They were companions and friends. The attachment of owner and dog is critical to the success of their relationship, and a guide dog also fulfills the role of a companion.

Like most dogs, a guide dog is a social lubricant or magnet for social interaction; this is probably not news to anyone who has regularly walked their own dog through a neighborhood and found that their neighbors know their dog's name but not theirs. Frank noted that while strangers he met might not know how to approach him—they just did not know how to converse with a blind person—Buddy opened the door to meet people, as they would comment on his beautiful dog. For anyone who lives in isolation from blindness or disability, opening up social connections is an essential aspect of quality of life, and Frank found it so.

Buddy was serious about her work and enjoyed an active and interesting social life. Buddy was fond of cats. She and the resident cat at Seeing Eye, Inc. were friends. One time when the traveling pair returned home, the Seeing Eye, Inc. cat had kittens, and Buddy carefully picked one up and brought it to Frank. In his memoir, *First Lady of the Seeing Eye,* Frank wrote about an incident when Buddy and he were visiting a college, and the president of the college thoughtfully suggested that Buddy could take a romp through the beautiful campus. The German shepherd returned with a strange scent that wafted over to Frank as she rubbed her head against his trouser leg. She had come dashing back, and it was clear she had been visiting a "black and white cat" and had taken skunk spray right in the face. Everyone's clothes had to be hung out and laundered; Frank recalled how the smell lingered. After he had spent the night in the president's suite, he had to make an unanticipated change of quarters. He paid $10 to a veterinarian to have Buddy deodorized but could not find anyone to do the same service for him. For a month, wherever Frank went into a hotel room on a damp day, the bellhop would sniff and say he thought the room had an odd odor. Frank would always say: "Don't bother. I like the smell."[56]

As Buddy and Frank began traveling, Frank would have Buddy on the speaking platform with him as he presented the story of The Seeing Eye. Frank had to learn public speaking, but Buddy was a natural. Not being an experienced speaker, Frank would feel nervous in front of so many people as he spoke, but Buddy behaved "as if she had been born in a theatrical trunk, one of a backstage litter."[57] She stood straight and alert, with her intelligent eyes beaming with excitement. When the person introducing Frank completed the introduction and said Frank's name, the audience applauded, and Buddy would join in with rousing barks. The audience loved it. Frank and Buddy traveled 5,000 miles and even visited the White House and President Calvin Coolidge.

Buddy enjoyed travel. Riding in the car, the beautiful German shepherd would assume an elegant position, with a paw draped over the handrest and eyes looking straight ahead as copilot. She took great interest in everything they passed and apparently expected everyone in the car to do so. Frank reported that on one excursion, a young woman was riding in the back seat with Buddy after a long Seeing Eye meeting. After looking at her dozing companion a few minutes, Buddy pushed her own wet nose over to the sleeping woman and knocked the sleepy lady's hat off as if to say, "People who see can enjoy the privilege."[58]

When it came to a young man's monumental challenge of understanding women, Buddy lent a female touch; she helped demystify the dating arena for Frank. She seemed to be able to pick the ideal partner for the evening— or so her blind handler thought. Frank also looked to Buddy to determine what kind of date a woman might prefer—bright lights or a quiet evening at home. When a date and Frank stopped by his room for a cocktail, if Buddy took her usual place on his bed, Frank assumed that Buddy could tell the girl wanted to spend an evening on the town. On the occasion when Buddy reclined on the sofa or the chair, to Frank that meant a cozy evening at home was the order of the evening.

Buddy developed a good sense of timing about when to speak up. The skill came in handy. On one occasion, she barked and chased a house burglar; in another case, when a thief with a gun approached Frank with a demand for money, Buddy stood still and did not attack. She had watched police dogs being trained back in Switzerland and knew guns meant danger.

Buddy and Frank worked as a team in some unusual ways. Swimming was a favorite for Buddy. She and Frank, accompanied by Frank's girlfriend, went to a lake to enjoy a day of swimming. Rubber bathing suits were the fashion, and Frank's date was wearing one. Buddy liked to paddle from one swimmer to another and would greet them by putting her paws on the person's shoulders. The girl was not expecting the attention, and Buddy inadvertently moved away unexpectedly, ripping her bathing suit from top to bottom. Buddy and Frank had to go back to the house to retrieve a towel so his girl could leave the water without being exposed. Frank recalled that it was very unfair he was blind, as he was unable to enjoy the situation thoroughly.[59] Buddy had been an unwitting accomplice.

Frank shared a touching realization in his autobiography: "The knowledge to meet unusual circumstances comes not from the dog training school's curriculum but from the dog's desire to care for his master or mistress stemming from their mutual love."[60] He realized that being blind, he could never fully realize all that Buddy did for him unless a sighted person was present to tell him of her exploits. He was not aware of all the obstacles she helped him avoid and the hazards he never knew existed. As one example, as he came to a streetcar toward home one day he gave her the command left. She would not turn; she wanted to go straight ahead into the street. He heard the dogs and children, so he thought she wanted to go over and say hello. He repeated it, she responded, and he banged right into a steamer truck. He knew then he should have listened to what his dog was trying to tell him.

Buddy gave Frank more than mobility; she gave him the courage to do things he never dreamed he would be able to do. He would have lacked the courage to ask a girl to become his wife in his helpless "pre–Buddy" state, and he said he possibly would not have wanted the type of girl who would have accepted. "She would want to mother me. I lived as a free, independent, and confident bachelor, and the only girl I could love is one who knew I could take care of myself." Frank met and married his wife, Lois, and stated that she "has never allowed me to blame no action on blindness."[61]

The Seeing Eye in America

Dorothy Eustis and Morris Frank capitalized on Buddy's success to help in recruiting sponsors for a dog guide training school in America. The team needed and found good staff candidates, both dogs, and people. In 1929, The Seeing Eye Incorporated was founded in Nashville, Tennessee, the first person-dog school in the United States. The Seeing Eye offered dog training, instructor training, housing, and training of person-dog teams. As The Seeing Eye graduated students and dogs who returned to their communities across the United States, publicity about their work spread and they became in high demand for speaking engagements around the country. Frank eventually became the operating manager of The Seeing Eye and Buddy traveled the country as the first trained guide dog in the United States.

The success of The Seeing Eye in America encouraged Eustis to set up another guide dog school in Vevey, Switzerland, in 1928. Two years afterward, in 1931, the Guide Dog for the Blind Association was started in the United Kingdom. Since then, guide dog schools have opened around the world, and new ones continue to open. They work for increased mobility, independence, and dignity of blind and partially sighted people.[62]

The summers were too hot in Nashville, so the school eventually relocated to Whippany, New Jersey, in 1941, and then to Morristown, New Jersey, in 1965, where it remains today. In 1979, they began breeding labs, golden retrievers, and lab mixes. After the Japanese attacked Pearl Harbor, the board of trustees of The Seeing Eye decided that the Seeing Eye dogs would be provided at no cost to those who had lost their sight in the line of duty, and Frank with Buddy II toured military facilities to support this effort.[63]

Dorothy Eustis retired as president of The Seeing Eye in 1940.[64] Buddy died of cancer in 1938. The first Buddy was the first of six Seeing Eye dogs that Frank had; all were named Buddy. Frank retired from The Seeing Eye in 1956, at age 48, to found his own insurance agency in Morristown.

When the Seeing Eye, Inc. celebrated its 500th graduation, 2,600 people had come through the program.[65] The mission of the Seeing Eye today remains "to enhance the independence, dignity, and self-confidence of people who are blind through the use of specially trained Seeing Eye dogs."[66] The program continues to breed, raise, and train Seeing Eye dogs; it instructs blind people in the proper care and training of a Seeing Eye dog and conducts and supports research in canine health and development.[67] Four primary breeds are used today for breeding: German shepherds, Labrador retrievers, golden retrievers, and Labrador/golden retriever crosses. Standard poodles are trained for persons with allergies. Instructor apprentices spend several months as kennel assistants, progress to initial obedience training, and then receive dogs of their own to teach—a process that typically takes four months.[68] Most of the training methods initially used by Humphrey are still in practice today at The Seeing Eye.

Legacy: Access and Independence

> I would rather walk with a friend in the dark than alone in the light.
> —Heller Keller[69]

ACCESS

Frank, Buddy, and The Seeing Eye fought successfully to help blind persons with guide dogs gain access to public places. Guide dogs and their handlers had to deal with problems of inaccessibility. Restaurants and other public places still refused dogs, and trains required dogs to ride in baggage cars, which defeated the purpose of their assistance role. Americans were still dubious about Seeing Eye dogs being everywhere. Laws about dogs related to the dangers dogs pose, such as the potential spread of rabies or killing livestock. No-pet policies became popular and having a guide dog created the need for an exception to the no-pets rule.[70]

Morris Frank, in his role as The Seeing Eye's vice president, traveled throughout the United States and Canada to communicate the need for equal access laws for people with guide dogs and to share the work of The Seeing

Eye. Frank championed the right to be accompanied by his guide dog. By 1956, every state in the country had passed laws guaranteeing blind people with guide dogs access to public spaces.[71]

Today, guide dogs are the most protected assistance dog in the world.[72] Federal and state laws provide access for guide dogs.[73] Guide, hearing, and service dogs are permitted, by the Americans with Disabilities Act, to accompany a person with a disability almost anywhere the public is allowed, including restaurants, businesses, and airplanes. With these rights also come responsibilities. Service animals are defined as dogs that are individually trained to do work or perform tasks for people with disabilities, which includes guide dogs for the blind.[74] The work that the dog has been trained to do must be directly related to the person's disability. Assistance dogs are considered working animals, not pets.

RESEARCH AND STUDY

Buddy and Frank's relationship and work inspired learning and research that continues today about the relationship between guide dogs and their owners. Humans learn from dogs in many ways, and guide dog teams teach us about the human-animal bond, about our relationship with and responsibilities toward working dogs, and about ourselves.

Today The Seeing Eye, Inc., is a place of learning and study about guide dog-human relationships.[75] A study conducted at The Seeing Eye, Inc., in 2017 found that "helicopter parents"[76] did not make for future guide dog success. Rather, "tough love" was an element in the raising of successful guide dogs. Emily Bray and a group of researchers studied long-term effects of maternal styles, observing 23 mothers and 98 puppies for the first five weeks.[77] The goal was to differentiate how the mothers interacted with puppies regarding the nursing position, time looking away, and time nearby licking and grooming the pups. After tracking the puppies for two years, they found that those whose moms were more attentive were less likely to graduate as a guide dog. This finding seems to suggest that dogs that had to work harder or overcome obstacles have more skills for success and for overcoming obstacles. The researchers concluded that more research was needed to continue to refine methods to identify successful guide dog candidates. The information on parenting techniques and helicopter parenting has generated interest in other areas.[78] The study is an example of how we can learn from interspecies behavior to understand both species.

Other studies on the human–guide dog relationship continue to increase the knowledge about human and guide dog collaboration in the spirit of the relationship between Morris Frank and Buddy, the first American guide dog. Knowledge about the successful matching of a blind person with a guide dog is important. Research and study can help identify critical matching aspects or identify problems early. An unsuccessful partnership can result in reduced mobility and quality of life for a usually impaired person and is also difficult for the dog. Since time and money are required to train guide dogs, it is essential to know what makes a successful guide dog-human partnership.

Lloyd and others also studied successful and unsuccessful guide dog matching and concluded that understanding what makes a successful partnership in guide dog-handler relationships is increasingly important, as there has been a steady increase in the number of handler-guide dog teams graduating around the world and in the number of other service or assistance animals.[79] The success of the relationship between them is dependent on both parties, not just the dog or person alone.[80] The researchers noted that the transition from one dog to another was recurring, that guide dog owners may experience the end of the dog relationship more times than the average owner, and retiring a guide dog may be difficult for not only the owner but for family and friends and for the dog. Nicholson and others identified distress arising from the end of a guide dog partnership. The ending of the relationship is especially painful to the owner, mainly when the dog has special significance to the owner, is his or her first dog, or the partnership ends abruptly. Emotions at the loss of the dog may be similar to those following the death of a pet, the death of a loved one, or the loss of sight.[81]

Seeing Eye dogs serve as guides, so they must exhibit sophisticated skills such as impulse control, flexible attention, and independent problem-solving. The Seeing Eye conducted a puppy development study in collaboration with the University of Pennsylvania. A Penn psychology graduate student, assisted by three Penn undergraduates, spent time at the Breeding Facility and at Stabile Canine Health Center. They followed a group of 137 pups from birth to completion of The Seeing Eye program. The study included behavioral testing and analysis of cortisol levels in the saliva of the dogs. Each puppy's early experiences, behavioral differences, and personalities over time were studied, and a biostatistician compiled and analyzed the extensive information. It is the goal of the study to improve our understanding of behavioral development regarding temperament and cognition. Collaborations such as this one are important as The Seeing Eye continues to strive to provide the best dogs to returning graduates and new students.[82]

A study by Craigon and others in 2017 revealed that the dog's safe behavior in the face of traffic was the most important positive aspect of a guide dog's behavior. Pulling the harness was the most discussed negative aspect of guide dog behavior.[83] Owners cited several significant issues, including distraction, eagerness and willingness, obedience, interaction with the public, and stress resistance—with attentiveness, obedience, confidence, and consistency rated as most important. The hardest part of having a guide dog,

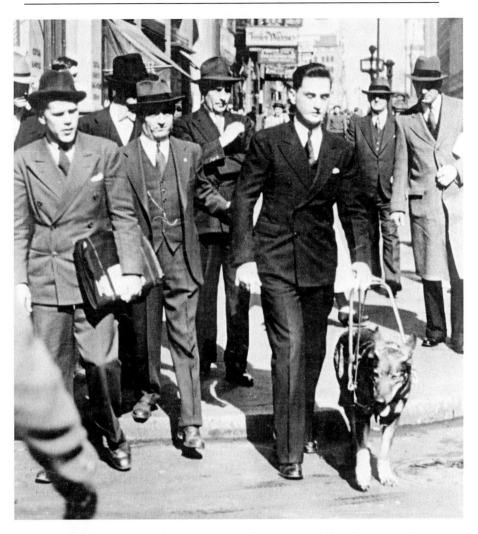

Morris Frank and his guide dog Buddy cross a busy New York City Street, 1928 (courtesy The Seeing Eye, Inc.).

according to the study, was public interference with the dog. Interference takes the form of grabbing the dog or trying to assist when not asked to do so by grabbing the dog or the harness.

A Pioneer to Light the Darkness

Buddy walked in the darkness with Morris Frank, and together they lit up America and opened up a new frontier for those who could not see. Since

1929, more than 17,000 partnerships of Seeing Eye dogs and humans have been established throughout the world. Today an average of 260 new teams are trained each year at The Seeing Eye, Inc., in Morristown, and an estimated 1,700 Seeing Eye dog teams are living in the United States and Canada.[84] Over 300 presentations are made each year to public groups representing The Seeing Eye.

Morris Frank and his wife traveled for several years throughout the United States sharing the work of The Seeing Eye, Inc., and Buddy. In 1984, Frank's autobiography, *First Lady of The Seeing Eye,* was made into a movie, *Love Leads the Way.* Morris Frank was invited to meet with several U.S. presidents. On the 75th anniversary of the school's founding, a bronze statue of Morris Frank and Buddy, entitled "The Way to Independence," was dedicated in Morris Frank Park, Morristown, New Jersey.[85]

Buddy, and the guide dogs that followed her, helped America see what disabled persons can accomplish and showed us the value of interspecies collaboration. She was a guide, companion, inspiration, and teacher to a generation of blind persons who came out of the darkness to the light at the other end of the leash. Buddy was a first in America. She blazed a trail at the side of Morris Frank.

Morris Frank expressed Buddy's legacy best. "She was a real pioneer as surely as others who discovered and brought ideas and lands to the New World. She discovered a new world for the blind."[86]

6

Jingles and Boris Levinson: Cotherapists

The doorbell rang unexpectedly. Psychologist Boris Levinson walked to the door, and his dog Jingles followed him. Jingles sat at Levinson's feet while the child psychologist wrote at his desk, but it was unusual for the dog to be in the office during the day. Jingles was not allowed in Levinson's office when he expected his young patients, but this morning the child and parent had arrived an hour before the appointment time.

Levinson opened the office door to find a distraught mother and her young son. They had arrived several hours early for an appointment they had made with Levinson to see if he would take the boy on as a patient. The child had already been through a long series of unsuccessful treatments and was showing increasing signs of withdrawal; hospitalization was a possibility.

When Levinson greeted the mother, Jingles ran to the boy. The dog leaped up and began to lick the young patient. Levinson saw the boy cuddle up to Jingles and start to pet him. The psychologist was surprised that the child did not shrink from the dog. The mother approached to stop the boy from petting Jingles, but Levinson encouraged her to let the interaction continue. Levinson allowed Jingles to remain in the room for the rest of the interview. After some time, the boy asked if Jingles always played with children who came to Levinson's office. When Levinson answered yes, the child asked to return for another session to play with Jingles.

The boy became Levinson's patient, and as the therapy proceeded, the child continued to play with Jingles. At first, Levinson noticed that his patient did not seem to be aware of the doctor's presence. The child focused only on the dog, although the young patient still listened and responded to Levinson's questions. Eventually, some of the affection the boy had for the dog spilled over to Levinson. The boy invited the psychologist to join in the play with Jingles. Levinson was slowly able to establish a rapport, and therapeutic relationship with the boy.[1]

Levinson credited the eventual rehabilitation of the child to Jingles, whom he called his cotherapist.[2] Levinson began working with Jingles with other patients.

Eight years later, Boris Levinson stood before his colleagues at the 1962 annual convention of the American Psychological Association in New York City. He presented his findings on working with Jingles.[3] His colleagues laughed, joked and asked if Jingles shared in Levinson's fees.[4] While some of his colleagues were enthusiastic, most were skeptical, responding to Jingles' story with guffaws and, in some cases, downright derision.

It was the era of the Beatles, Woodstock, civil rights, moon shots, and social change. However, in 1962, the psychological community was not ready to consider a new therapeutic approach—that a dog could have a significant role in psychotherapeutic treatment. Levinson's psychological colleagues had not begun to explore the science of interspecies comfort and healing. Animals in a therapeutic role were a new and disconcerting concept to them. Most of them ridiculed and belittled Levinson's findings. That was about to change.

The story of Jingles and Levinson is one of the most famous stories in the history of animal-assisted therapy and the human-animal bond.[5] Levinson had demonstrated that companion animals can help to form a strong connection between patient and therapist.[6] It was a pioneer's journey of a man and his dog, and Levinson gave full credit to his dog Jingles. He said that his discovery of the "use of a dog as an accessory in the treatment of disturbed children" came inadvertently through Jingles' own intervention.[7]

However, Levinson's colleagues were uncomfortable talking about the role of animals as collaborators in psychotherapy. Levinson felt that the reason some therapists objected to the use of the dog in a therapeutic setting was the anxiety clinicians and other humans had because of our relationship with the nonhuman environment.[8] Others such as Carl Rogers[9] felt that the anxiety was related to resistance to a new psychotherapeutic technique. His colleagues' ridicule of Levinson may have been in response to their own discomfort. Still, some were intrigued and began to consider the possibility of human-animal integration in psychology.[10]

Stanley Coren, Ph.D., a psychology professor, and researcher at the University of British Columbia in Vancouver, was present during Levinson's 1962 presentation and recalled his firsthand experience of the reaction. Coren, writing in his online series "Canine Corner" in *Psychology Today,*[11] recalled that Levinson presented the findings from his work and that the reception of the conference attendees was not positive. Coren doubted he would hear much more about the use of animals in a therapeutic environment.[12] As it turned out, Levinson and Jingles would receive help from an unexpected source—a dog pioneer of the past, Jofi.

Levinson's presentation came about 15 years after the death of Sigmund Freud, and several new biographies had been released that included letters and translations of his books and journals. Many of the biographies, some written by individuals who actually knew Freud, featured Jofi, Freud's chow, and her role in and around the couch of the father of psychoanalysis. Many biographers indicated that Jofi was a feature in Freud's life and in his psychoanalytical technique and revealed that Freud considered his dog an adjunct therapeutic partner, a cotherapist of sorts. Jofi's presence in Freud's consulting room and her role in the analysis process lent legitimacy to the place of a dog in the psychotherapeutic setting.[13] Even the most skeptical of Levinson's psychologist colleagues were reluctant to doubt that a dog could be a worthy therapeutic partner if the great Freud occasionally enlisted a four-legged assistant.

While the psychological community was initially reluctant to accept the premise of Levinson's description of a dog as a cotherapist, therapists were actually using animals in their practices. In 1972, Levinson reported that he and his colleagues sampled 50 percent of the membership of the Clinical Division of the New York State Psychological Association about the extent to which pets were recommended by the therapists as aids to therapy. Of the 319 respondents, 33 percent indicated that they had used pets as therapeutic adjuncts to their treatment, and 91 percent found them useful.[14]

Jingles: Canine Cotherapist

We are able to get to know Jingles through a review of Boris Levinson's writing. Just as Freud had noted in his work with Jofi, Levinson noted that when Jingles joined him in the therapy room, the dog facilitated therapeutic communication. Levinson found that after first developing a relationship with Jingles, his young patients went on to develop a relationship with the therapist.

Levinson began studying the effects of dog-assisted psychotherapy, gathering data, writing, and presenting his findings. In 1962, he published his paper "The Dog as a 'Co-therapist'"[15] in the journal *Mental Hygiene*. Levinson wrote the paper eight years after first working with Jingles in his practice. "The Dog as a 'Co-therapist'" was the first paper in the professional literature to present the therapeutic possibility of the human-animal bond. Levinson's paper laid the foundation for future research in animal-assisted therapy. In a second article in 1964,[16] Levinson first used the term *pet therapy*.

Levinson's papers and books explained his approach in pet therapy and explained that pets could be useful in two ways: as psychotherapeutic aides in the therapist's office and as adjuncts for therapy in the home of emotionally disturbed children.[17] In 1969, Levinson published his book *Pet-Oriented Child Psychotherapy*. Writing in this landmark book, Boris Levinson explained again that it was the initiative of his dog Jingles that "played the leading role in what proved to be a most startling drama."[18] As Jofi had done in Freud's consulting room, Jingles stepped into Levinson's consultations and demonstrated the benefits of the human-animal connection. Levinson described his discovery with Jingles as "accidental."[19]

Boris Levinson

A psychoanalytically trained psychologist, Levinson was a professor of psychology at Yeshiva University in New York, a diplomate in clinical psychology, and a member of the American Board of Examiners in Professional Psychology. He had a Ph.D. in clinical psychology from New York University.[20] He was born in 1907 in Lithuania and came to the United States in 1923 with his family; he became a naturalized citizen in 1930. In 1972, he retired from Yeshiva University and assumed a position as director of the human/companion animal therapy program at the Blueberry Treatment Center in Brooklyn, New York, a center for autistic children.[21]

Levinson was a prolific writer with broad interests. His research interests included exploring new techniques and approaches to helping disturbed children. He understood that the path to introducing pets in therapy would not be easy, and his ideas might not be accepted, but he persisted. When Levinson first experienced his "accidental" discovery provided by Jingles' initiative, he first rejected any thought of pursuing the subject further because it seemed too "unorthodox."[22] He decided to present his findings and theory at the New York conference because he felt he was willing to modify existing therapeutic principles if it were to benefit patients.

Levinson had a generous spirit. He believed that too many children were in need with too few therapists, and pets might be a way to decrease the long treatment time. He felt that something very significant occurred when a child played with a pet yet did not utter a single word. He professed, "Healing ... sometimes does occur in the most unexpected places."[23] Levinson believed that, in certain clinical situations, a pet could become part of the treatment plan. This was revolutionary indeed in an already skeptical profession.

In his writings, Levinson described the principles of his work and how pets had many benefits, especially for a disturbed child. Levinson felt the dog "can be and often is a companion, friend, servant, admirer, confidante, slave, scapegoat, a mirror of trust or a defender for the child." Levinson held that "when a child needs to love safely without fear of losing the love object, and without losing face, a dog can provide this."[24] A dog provides a safe, nonjudgmental affectionate relationship with a child and can't talk back when yelled at by a child; the child can do no wrong."[25] Levinson explained that this is important for disturbed children because they do not want to be judged but want to be accepted and permitted to have symptoms without their loved ones criticizing or creating feelings of guilt.

Jingles was crucial to the therapeutic work, in that when the dog was present, the child was now master and could order Jingles about; the dog was now the child's friend and ally and not the therapist's. Although Levinson worked with several dogs, Jingles was the only one he identified by name in his writing. Levinson's writing did not describe Jingles or tell us what breed Jingles was, but he wrote of his affection and gratitude to the dog.

Levinson introduced Jingles selectively with certain children. He integrated standard questions about pets into his assessment interviews. Jingles served as a cotherapist as Levinson looked to Jingles for clues for what the child was struggling with or problems the child was having difficulty expressing. The children would begin to respond to someone outside themselves. Levinson's experience with Jingles provided the inspiration and encouragement for him to pursue the study of how to use animals in the treatment of withdrawn children.

Jingles: Healing in Unexpected Places

By most of Levinson's accounts, Jingles was a canine extrovert and was enthusiastic about the work. Jingles made his canine presence known by nuzzling for affection and engaging in play. In the therapy session, Jingles elicited a wide range of responses from young patients. Jingles' presence, especially on a first visit, made the session seem less threatening. His dog bowl, food, and dog toys were often present in the room.

Like most therapy dogs, Jingles' role in the therapy setting was to encourage young patients to accept themselves, to create a feeling of safety, and to encourage children to communicate and share feelings. In her book, *Why the Wild Things: Animals in the Lives of Children*, Gail F. Melson explored how animals affect children's lives and how animals can be therapeutic and educational for children. She described Levinson's work with Jingles at Blueberry Center and how a friendly dog in a therapy session could help create a feeling of safety for young patients, and especially for highly withdrawn children.[26] Levinson was known as both a rigorous academician and a man who was warm and loving with children. One colleague at the Blueberry Center commented, "He came to Blueberry every day with Jingles, but the children did not call the dog Jingles; they all called him Levinson. They loved Grandpa Boris."[27]

Levinson wrote about Jingles' role in the dynamics of the pet therapy process. One of the primary functions played by Jingles was to ease the anxiety involved with meeting a therapist. Through play with a dog in the session, a child could rehearse and try to resolve some of life's problems.

In the beginning, the patient just talked and petted Jingles and involved Jingles in imaginative play. Jingles didn't really participate but just allowed the child to handle him. The child paid no attention to the therapist at this point. The next stage of the therapy might involve Jingles as the center of the child's fantasy and activity, and Jingles might be directed by the child to participate in the imagined play scenario. Levinson might be an accessory to the session at this point. Later, the child might engage in other activities in which the dog participated but played a role subsidiary to that of the therapist. At this point in the therapy, Jingles was not the central partner in the therapeutic exchange, which occurred between the therapist and child. Some children would find it easier to accept affection from a pet than from an adult. Because many of Levinson's young patients could not tolerate monotony and had an inner restlessness created by their emotional turmoil, they might be embarrassed by their lack of control. They welcomed the addition of a canine companion who was often just as restless as they were. Levinson might say Jingles wants to do this or that or point out that the dog wanted to explore every nook and cranny of the therapist's office.[28]

Levinson explained that the process for introducing a child to Jingles automatically standardized itself. It began with the child playing with the dog and asking Jingles to shake hands and dance. A cookie might be offered to Jingles as an incentive. Sometimes children who felt undeserving of any kindness would hesitate to ask Levinson to share something with them. But these children did not hesitate to remark "Jingles is hungry" or "The dog wants to eat." The child might raid the refrigerator and prepare a meal that the dog, the therapist, and the child could enjoy together. Often children made a ritual for the preparation of the meal. It seemed important for the children to establish that the dog was the child's friend and not the therapist's.[29]

"I Am Jingles"

Levinson reported a therapeutic anecdote in which the child shook hands with Jingles and danced with the dog. Levinson gave Jingles a cookie as a reward. Then the child said, "I am Jingles. I also want to dance." The child got down on the floor, howled like a wolf, asked Levinson to give him a cookie, and inquired, "Why can't you have two dogs and can't you take me as one of them?"[30] He asked Levinson about his wife and his children. Levinson interpreted this as the child wanting to become part of the therapist's family, with the child volunteering: "If the human component of your family is full, the dog component is not, and he would like to be considered if a vacancy existed."[31]

From Levinson's descriptions, it appears that Jingles accomplished his role as a therapy dog just by being himself. Anyone who has spent any amount of time around dogs can appreciate that they can be curious and spontaneous. However, dogs will be dogs. They scratch when they itch, and they live in the moment. It is up to their handler to help them socialize in appropriate ways. Corrections and education are often necessary—even for experienced therapy dogs and adult humans. This process of correction also became part of the pet-assisted psychotherapy learning for a child. Children might identify with Jingles—a dog who messes up and could just be himself and still be loved.

Jingles accomplished his role by behaving as dogs will. He might do some licking or create an occasional mess or not follow instructions—and this opportunity gave the child a sense of "I guess if Jingles is not always good and we still like him, I might not be so bad."[32] Levinson held that children with psychological issues want to be accepted and admired without being berated for transgressions or made to feel guilty. They have an intense need to matter to someone who accepts them no matter what. With a dog, children have the enriching experience of complete mutual acceptance. Even if a dog defecates or engages in public and indiscriminate sexual activity, he is loved and accepted. The child makes comparisons. If the dog doesn't feel guilty, why should the child?[33]

Levinson reported a case scenario in which a family dog had chewed the family's best shoes and that the child noted that the dog was loved regardless of what he did. At one time, a patient's pet dog had been brought to Levinson's office and had diarrhea during the session, and the patient's mother cleaned it up. A crucial time in the patient's treatment came when the child realized she could learn to accept her own "badness," that she too could mess up and still be loved.[34]

Jingles, the child, and the therapist observing the interactions between dog and child became a living lab. Levinson could study the child's inner world by asking, "How does the child react to Jingles?" or asking the child "What do you think Jingles might be thinking?" The child might wonder about Jingles' ability to smell or hear things others couldn't. At this point, Levinson might discuss with the child how some people may perceive or feel things that others do not. This might lead to the child reflecting on his own feelings and whether they are as important to others as they are to him.[35]

Levinson felt that the use of a pet such as Jingles could be integrated into the treatment plan for the child. Levinson preferred the term "pet therapy" rather than "play therapy" because play therapy connoted a self-chosen activity absent the structured setting of a therapist's office.[36] Levinson differentiated between two types of pet therapy: one in which the therapist used an animal in the office and the one in which, as an aid to therapy, a pet was, in a directed way, introduced into the patient's home. Jingles functioned as an aid to therapy in the office. As far as we know, Jingles did not make home visits, although he did walk with patients in what Levinson called ambulation therapy. Taking the dog for a walk removed the therapy from the sterile environment of the consulting room and brought it into the larger laboratory of the outside world.

The fundamental intent of the techniques Levinson used with Jingles were to be therapeutic. Animal-assisted therapy is designed to achieve such goals as establishing the psychotherapeutic relationship, building rapport, role modeling, providing reassurance and a feeling of safety, and providing opportunities for role-playing, transference, and interpretation.[37] Additional intentions might be encouraging insight, facilitating social or relationship skills, enhancing self-confidence, and enhancing trust.[38] To accomplish these goals today a therapist might encourage the patient to pet, touch, play with, or hold the therapy animal during sessions or encourage the child to tell the dog about a problem, distress, or concern the patient was having. Taking the dog for a walk, teaching the dog a skill or trick, or getting the child to have the dog perform a command are other interventions. A therapist might encourage the child to make up stories about what the dog thinks about a subject, as Levinson did. Involving the dog or encouraging exploratory conversations can encourage the expression of feelings.

Levinson Calls for Research

The journey to that pioneering moment when Levinson stood before the American Psychological Association to introduce the role of a dog as a therapist had been a lengthy one. Although the therapeutic benefits of pets and animals had been noted as early as Florence Nightingale's work, there was still no scientific study of these efforts or their outcomes. The journey to acknowledge the therapeutic benefits of pets had begun as early as 1699 when John Locke advocated "giving children dogs, squirrels, birds or any such thing to look after as a means of encouraging them to develop tender feelings and a sense of responsibility toward others."[39] Farm animals were present at the York Quaker Retreat in England, founded in 1792, for the mental health benefit of patients. The Society of Friends started the retreat to encourage kind treatment of the mentally ill.[40] Some of the patients at the retreat cared for small animals to benefit by helping creatures more dependent than themselves, to occupy their time, and to "awaken social and benevolent feelings."[41] In 1867, farm animals were utilized to help patients at Bethel Center, a community in Germany.[42]

Animals were used as emotional support in the United States in 1919 when U.S. Secretary of Interior Franklin K. Lane brought dogs to socialize with patients at St. Elizabeth's Hospital in Washington, D.C., a federal psychiatric hospital. Later, dogs were present in the 1940s at an Air Force convalescent center in New York City.[43] On August 12, 1919, Secretary Lane wrote to Dr. William Alanson White, who was thought of at the time as "chief psychiatrist of the United States":

> Would it not be possible to have some dogs over there that the men could play with and chum with? If you could find friendly fellows like bulldogs, who look fierce and are gentle, or big noble fellows like Newfoundlands, I should think they would be great entertainment for the men. A poor insane chap naturally reaches for companionship and finds himself barred by the various limitations of his unfortunate associates, but he could develop a great friendship with a dog.[44]

White replied on August 18 that he would be glad to try it.[45]

At the U.S. Army Air Forces Convalescent Center in Pawling, New York, a rehabilitation center, patients worked with farm animals and cared for pet dogs.[46] Howard Archibald Rusk developed the Pawling program and is generally recognized as the "father of rehabilitative medicine."[47]

The journey for full acceptance of a dog in the therapy room would be long and filled with skepticism. Why did it take so long for animal-assisted therapy to enter the psychotherapist's treatment considerations? The practice of animals assisting in psychotherapy required a documented science and theory base to support its benefits. Levinson and Jingles were true pioneers, especially in Levinson's call for more scientific research on the benefits of animals in human health. Levinson understood the need for and encouraged the development of a body of theory, a methodology, and specific terms for the discipline. When Levinson and Jingles first demonstrated how pets could assist in psychotherapy, no scientific studies had been published on the benefits or impact of animals in psychiatric treatment.[48] In the 1960s, psychology and psychotherapy were evolving from Freudian theoretical frameworks to broader psychodynamic theories. Before Levinson's work, most psychoanalysts approached the use of dogs in therapy as symbols rather than considering how integrating the dog in the therapy would affect the patient.[49]

Levinson felt that the success he had with Jingles in therapy had broad mental hygiene implications, which the professional community could not overlook.[50] He also stressed the need for research to prove it. Twenty years after he first presented to the American Psychological Association, Levinson published comments on the future of research into relationships between people and their animal companions.[51] He concluded that, while the problems and issues raised in his original 1961 paper and his subsequent articles had come to be taken more seriously by the professional community and society at large, it seemed to him that the field of animal-human relationships had not yet become a true discipline[52] and scientific research was still meager.[53]

Levinson identified four main areas of focus for future investigation: the role of animals in various human cultures and ethnic groups over the centuries; the effect of the association of animals on human personality development; human-animal communication; and the therapeutic use of animals in formal psychotherapy, institutional settings, and residential arrangements for handicapped and aged populations.[54] He challenged clinicians to pursue critical and intriguing questions involving the human-animal cotherapist relationship. He challenged his colleagues to examine pet therapy as a tool that could promote emotional healing for children and to consider how the use of a pet in the therapeutic setting might affect the relationship between therapist and patient. He encouraged more study into questions of how the personalities of therapist and patient and animal interact, and what problems might lend themselves to resolution with animal-assisted play therapy. He encouraged research into how the use of a therapy animal compares with other therapies for the same issues and what kinds of animals would be most helpful to patients with specific types of difficulties.[55]

So the journey for a research base for animal-assisted interventions continued. Today clinicians and others still seek clarification: What is animal-assisted therapy? What does a therapy dog actually do? Answers to this question and our definitions have more often than not been descriptive and varied; they explain what the dogs do, but those explanations are not framed within a consistent, agreed-upon theoretical construct. However, the more we see therapy dogs in action, the more experience we have to study. As animal-assisted interventions become more popular and widespread decades after Levinson's work, definitions that are more precise have been proposed.

Legacy: A Dog as Cotherapist

As the 1960s generation ended, the emerging discipline of animal-assisted therapy was building upon the work of Dog Pioneers that had gone before. The breakthroughs accomplished by the Mercy Dogs, Nightingale's support of animals in healing, Jofi and Freud, and the training of guide dogs at Fortunate Fields had created curiosity about what the human-canine partnership could do to improve human health and health care.

Like Colonel Richardson's struggle to convince others of the value of ambulance dogs, Dr. Levinson's journey to persuade his colleagues that a dog could act as a cotherapist in child psychology required persistence and inspiration and its own set of trials. Fortunately, Levinson had a dog by his side and by the side of his young patients. His observations of Jingles provided the first empirical sharing of animal-assisted therapy with the professional community in spite of the skepticism it encountered.

Sigmund Freud and Jofi had demonstrated that a dog could be an asset and belonged in the psychoanalytical setting, and Levinson and Jingles broadened the role and demonstrated the need for the development of animal-human studies as a scientific discipline. Jingles and Jofi, two pioneering dogs guided by their human mentors, had crossed the threshold of psychological treatment to enter the treatment room as partners with humans. Jofi and Jingles inspired the work in earnest for empirical evidence to describe and measure the effects of the human-animal connection in mental health treatment. They were fortunate to have two human pioneers—Freud and Levinson—as mentors and partners who listened and paid attention.

Levinson also noted that research was needed into the best methods of training a dog for psychotherapeutic work, as well as training therapists to work in the new field. He noted the example provided at Fortunate Fields where they taught both the blind person and the dog, so the dog could get to know his handler and the person could get to know the dog's capabilities and possible handicaps.[56]

A new generation of clinicians and therapy dogs would soon pursue the quest for these answers. Today, mental health professionals who work with children are recognizing the value of animals as therapeutic adjuncts in treating issues such as loneliness or more complex issues such as autism. What was initially termed pet-assisted psychotherapy by Levinson is now redefined as animal-assisted therapy or animal-facilitated therapy. By any name, animals have found their way into the therapeutic process.[57]

Today, animal-assisted therapy has an increased presence in the scientific literature, with more interest in exploring it as a complementary intervention in mental health.[58] However, limited studies have been done with children and pediatric patients.[59] We needed pioneers like Jofi and Jingles to bring animal-assisted therapy and the human-animal connection to the office of the psychotherapist. We still need data and empirical evidence to support and understand animals' therapeutic benefit and how best to integrate trained therapy animals into mainstream care.

Jingles and Levinson brought the proof of the value of a dog in child psychiatry to the psychological community. Levinson documented his work with a dog as a therapeutic tool in working with child psychiatry. Levinson recalled that his first insight into the use of a dog as an accessory in the treatment of children came about accidentally. "It was my own dog Jingles who was to play a leading role in what proved to be a most startling drama."[60] Jingles so inspired Levinson that he dedicated his classic book, *Pet-Oriented Child Psychotherapy,* to him:

> This book is dedicated to Jingles, my co-therapist,
> To whom I owe more than he owes me;
> Who taught me more than I taught him;
> Who unveiled a completely new world of experience for me.[61]

Levinson and Jingles opened up new thinking and changed attitudes about the interconnectedness of human health and animals. Levinson understood that dogs and pets could teach us, not by becoming little humans, but by being themselves, being just plain "doggy." If we accept dogs as themselves, perhaps we can accept ourselves in all our messiness.

7

Boe and Budge: The First Combat and Operational Stress Control Dogs

The soldiers joked that their goal was to outrun the therapy dog in the 5K races.[1] When Sergeant First Class Boe, a female Labrador retriever, competed in the 5K race on the Iraq base, she was doing more than having fun. The combat and operational stress control (COSC) therapy dog was on duty on a serious mission—to boost morale in a community that needed a lift. Sergeant Boe's mission was to comfort, encourage, and support the mental health needs of the military community living on the base in Iraq.

Sergeants Boe and her partner Sergeant Budge, another deployed Labrador retriever, were great listeners. They had a knack for seeking out people who needed to talk. When a traumatic event occurs, sometimes soldiers or others affected want to talk about it. Sometimes they don't. Sometimes just petting and being near a dog helps.

Almost daily, a visitor to the therapy dogs would say "I just needed a hug" or, when the dog planted a sloppy kiss, would respond, "That is just what I needed!"[2] For soldiers far from home, a small gesture of unconditional love from a dog could make all the difference in the world.

Sergeant Boe and Sergeant Budge were the first COSC dogs to be deployed as specially trained therapy dogs in Iraq and Afghanistan.[3] The two therapy dogs were to work with the occupational therapists of the COSC unit. The dogs were to assist the COSC occupational therapist staff by breaking down barriers to seeking mental health services and facilitating social interaction between soldiers and occupational therapists.[4] Part of these canine soldiers' mission was to help reduce the stigma of seeking mental health services.

Part of the COSC therapy dogs' success resulted from the bond they formed in their new communities. Those bonds opened doors to boost morale and increase soldiers' motivation to talk with mental health professionals about tough issues.

Four-Legged Icebreakers

The COSC therapy dogs were great icebreakers. The therapy dogs and their handlers reached out to service members in their respective areas and offered counseling, classes, and command consultation. The work took the dogs to the gym, the dining room, and any place that presented an opportunity for interaction with the service community.[5] The COSC dog-handler team walked through hangers, motor pools, and work and living spaces to make contact and assess stress levels. The team's standard procedure was to introduce themselves, explain their services, and offer support.

Therapy dogs are utilized in goal-directed interventions working with a professional health care provider. An encounter with a therapy dog can often open the door to provide an opportunity for motivation, education, and recreational and therapeutic benefits to those reluctant to reach out for mental health services. The COSC therapy dogs turned out to be magnets for interaction between the occupational therapists and the soldiers. When the therapy dogs accompanied them, the occupational therapists were often approached by troops first.[6] Soldiers might ask about the dog's role in combat or share reminiscences of a pet at home. Many shared photos. When the COSC dog was present, service members seemed more likely to share their concerns, fears, and goals.

A friendly canine can open the door to communication for several reasons. Detachment from family often means separation from a companion animal as well as human family members. Adults who develop a significant attachment to pets can suffer considerable feelings of loss when they are away from home. A discussion about feelings of loss of a pet or other loss might open the door to discussing other issues and might lead to discussion of mental health services.

The soldiers were a group that may well have needed a "paw up." The largest demographic group in the military is 18 to 25 years old. These service members have been thought to have great potential to benefit from animal-assisted intervention since they may have had pets at home that they left when they went to serve in the military. Some of these young service members were away from home for the first time. Some were dealing with a variety of personal stresses. A therapy dog could make the counseling setting feel more homelike and could enhance communication.[7]

As the service members became more at ease with the COSC team, the dogs served as facilitators to move the service member into classes to assist with self-esteem, anger management, or communication skill building. One occupational therapist created a fitness plan for soldiers, and Boe ran with the soldier and even ran a 5K run on the base.[8] Participating in fitness events like the 5K run was part of being a good role model for human service members who were working on their fitness goals.

Besides making the therapists more approachable, the therapy dogs helped decrease the stigma of asking about mental health services, broke up the monotony of a deployment, and facilitated informing service members about available services. The therapist handlers noted that service members would talk to them for more extended periods of time with the dogs present. The dog's presence served as a lubricant for conversation. Therapy dogs might join the individual therapy session with the service member if requested and schedules permitted.

The dogs also helped with publicizing COSC services. Staff presented profiles and stories of the dogs on a flyer announcing their services. The handlers anecdotally noticed that more service member visits were scheduled when the flyer was posted. Service members tended to take more time to listen and learn about services available to the community.[9]

Boe and Budge became an integrated part of their communities and part of the military family. This built strong bonds with the troops and promoted trust, which facilitated access. The four-legged sergeants attended social events, parties, and celebrations. On her fourth birthday in October 2009, a party for Sergeant Boe was attended by more than 100 people. The party was for the dog, but it really was for the community.[10] The soldiers might not always remember the occupational therapist's name, but the COSC team would get invitations to events that mental health providers might not otherwise receive. Sergeant Budge was a charismatic favorite and sought-after guest at social gatherings in his community. Budge would often receive too many treats and had to receive smaller meals to control his weight.[11]

In 2009, Captain Brian Gregg was an army occupational therapist assigned to the COSC detachment, where he managed a clinic that provided behavioral health care for service members in Iraq. He conducted fitness and prevention operations and was assigned a COSC therapy dog partner, a tan Labrador retriever, Sergeant First Class Albert. Writing in a 2012 article,[12] Gregg provided an occupational therapist's perspective on animal-assisted therapy in a military environment. He gave a first-person account of the effect of reducing the stigma of attending stress reduction and anxiety prevention classes. Albert eased tension; he made soldiers more willing to seek out COSC for services and more open in discussing troubling issues. Albert enhanced the mood of clients as he engaged them as they entered the COSC clinic and during their appointments with providers. The therapy dog even visited soldiers at their duty station.

Gregg recalled that many clients, even those who did not have a love for dogs, would open up to the dog, and many would play fetch, pet him, and go through his series of commands. Albert assisted in classes, teaching life skills such as effective communication, assertiveness, and stress management. As the dog's popularity grew throughout the base population, Albert added units and clients to his weekly visits. Gregg described Albert as a "friend in an unforgiving environment."[13]

COSC Dog: New Role for a Military Dog

Dogs have served in mental health services in a variety of roles since the late 18th century when animals were incorporated into mental health institutions to increase socialization among patients.[14] The Mercy Dogs of World War I who had gone before had shown that a dog could comfort a dying soldier in the trenches. World War II saw dogs emerge in therapeutic roles to assist service members' recovery.[15] The use of human-animal interaction for therapy began in the United States in St. Elizabeth's Hospital in Washington, D.C. By World War II, the ability of dogs to help soldiers recover was starting to be recognized.

In her book *War Dogs: Tales of History, Heroism, and Love*, Rebecca Frankel described roles of military dogs in helping soldiers. She described an Associated Press report from the Anzio beachhead in Italy about a dog named Lulabelle. The tiny dog made rounds with chaplain Colonel William E. King in a hospital tent.[16] Lulabelle fit in the chaplain's pocket.[17]

Frankel described how a Red Cross volunteer at the Army Air Forces Convalescence Center in Pawling thought a dog might cheer up a recuperating soldier with a severely injured leg. A German shepherd puppy named Fritz was given to the soldier, and the soldier's recovery was so improved that soon other patients were asking for dogs. Two years later, Pawling installed an 80-foot kennel ready to house 50 dogs.[18]

Also in World War II, Smoky, a tiny Yorkshire terrier, became an early therapy dog helping comfort wounded soldiers in the same hospital where her handler, William Wynne, was hospitalized. Smoky became famous for helping comfort wounded soldiers. The underfed and scrawny dog had been discovered in a foxhole, and Wynne bought her from a friend. Wynne taught her tricks. One of her best tricks was to play dead for the wounded soldiers she visited. Wynne would point one finger at her, and she would fall to the ground and remain there limp even when he lifted her up. She developed a repertoire of tricks. When Wynne was hospitalized at the 233rd Station House for an illness, the commanding office permitted Smoky to visit and sleep with Wynne. One day, one of the nurses asked if she could bring Smoky around to visit the other battle-weary wounded, and Smoky was a hit. During the day, she visited recovering soldiers, who would laugh at her tricks. Wynne and Smoky were invited to visit other hospitals, and Smoky's reputation as an early therapy dog began. Smoky went on to distinguish herself in battle and became a war hero and a public figure.[19]

As awareness of the healing and comforting work of dogs with wounded soldiers increased, so did the trend of allowing dogs to visit wounded soldiers. Just as owners had volunteered their dogs to serve overseas in World War I, by 1947, civilians donated dogs to help cheer up wounded World War II soldiers.[20]

In the 1960s, when Boris Levinson introduced his concept of the dog as cotherapist in his psychotherapy with children, the psychological community began to become more convinced of the benefits of the animals in psychotherapeutic work.[21] An increasing number of programs in the United States slowly began to involve therapy dogs in their mental health services in some capacity.

In 1985, as army veterinarians studied the human-animal bond to determine ways it might contribute to military medicine, their interest and efforts provided a foundation on which later military efforts were based.[22] An animal-assisted program was in place at some army medical centers; it was supported by the local army medical commands and operated with a core group of Red Cross volunteers. The primary purpose of these programs was to "bring smiles to the patients, family members, and hospital staff." It was hoped that interacting and focusing on the dog might alleviate fear, anxiety, or pain.[23]

In 2007, a new role for dogs in the military operational environment began as Boe and Budge, now a pair of specially trained COSC dogs prepared to be deployed to Iraq and Afghanistan with the COSC unit. The dog's role was to break down perceived barriers and facilitate social interaction between soldiers and occupational health medical professionals who were the dog's handlers. Sergeants Boe and Budge went with the trained COSC units; they worked with the COSC and its teams and became an essential modality in the army's initiative to safeguard soldiers' mental health. It was therapy dogs' first use in COSC units.[24]

The initiative began when America's VetDogs was invited to train a dog to work with vestibular patients who were adjusting to a new prosthesis at Walter Reed Medical Center. A golden retriever named George was assigned to the job at Walter Reed. George's handler was eventually reassigned, but George had begun providing emotional support to service members and became a roving goodwill ambassador for recovering veterans. George had inspired thinking about a new role for therapy dogs who might be able to help break down the stigma that often prevented military members from seeking mental health assistance. In 2007, the U.S. Army Veterans Command consulted with the army surgeon general to discuss a proposal to send the two therapy dogs with COSC to America's VetDogs in Smithtown, New York. In December 2007, the army initiated the new program. Labrador retrievers, Boe and Budge, were donated and trained by America's VetDogs and were sent to New York for training with two occupational therapists. America's VetDogs is a not-for-profit organization that began as a program of the Guide Dog Foundation for the Blind. Today, the organization's goal is to provide enhanced mobility and independence to veterans, active-duty military, and first responders with disabilities. VetDogs places guide dogs for blind persons and those with low vision, as well as hearing dogs, physical and occupational therapy dogs that aid in rehabilitation, and post-traumatic stress disorder service dogs.[25]

Boe and Budge and the COSC dogs that followed them were therapy dogs, not service dogs. It is important to understand the distinction in their roles, scope of practice, responsibilities, and privileges. In military and civilian settings, different rules apply to service dogs and therapy dogs.[26] The primary distinction between assistance or service animals and therapy animals is that therapy animals, working under the direction of their handlers, provide services to persons with or without disabilities through the human-animal bond. An assistance dog is an animal supporting people who have disabilities. Assistance dogs are also commonly called service dogs. An assistance dog has been individually trained to do work or perform tasks for an individual with a disability.

Therapy animals are trained to assist a health care professional or allied health professional within the scope of a therapeutic treatment plan. Occupational therapists and other professionals use a therapy dog to help with obtaining treatment goals. A therapist may use a therapy dog to encourage an atmosphere of trust and acceptance during therapy sessions. Unlike assistance animals, therapy animals have no special rights of access, except in those facilities where they are welcomed.

Before the COSC dogs deployed, both dogs and their handlers received training. Although one person became the dog's primary handler, three others were also trained to ensure that staffing changes would not affect the dog's care. Training occurred at both the training camps and the unit's home base to train dogs' primary and secondary handlers. The dogs were trained by navigating different types of surfaces, busy streets, and highways. In addition to basic obedience training, they were exposed to varying kinds of vehicles, equipment, sights, and smells using a volunteer fire department near the VetDogs training facility. Firefighters might sound horns and flashlights so the dog's reaction could be assessed; a dog who bolted or showed fear would not be a candidate for the COSC program. Minor anxiety would not exclude a dog. Dogs were loaded and unloaded into a variety of vehicles. Trainers gently encouraged anxious dogs; the dogs were well acclimated to the sounds of gunfire from automatic weapons and the sounds of helicopters and other aircraft. Successfully trained dogs were able to behave well in a variety of situations. They had to be physically fit and were taught to ignore food distractions.[27]

The dogs had to be able to demonstrate sufficient energy for long hours and active work, such as providing emotional support and comfort through interactions such as playing fetch or physical activity. The dogs had to be able to adapt to multiple handlers due to the deployment of team members. All dogs needed to have veterinarian clearance because of the variety of conditions they would face and had to be screened for temperament and adaptability. The weather and conditions would be challenging, so the dogs had protective gear—booties to protect their paws and goggles to protect from blowing sand. They also had cooling jackets for daytime and warm vests for the night. When the dogs were fully trained, they were deployed to their assignment in the war zone.

The Mission

When troops are sent to a combat environment, the U.S. Army's COSC teams provide behavioral health treatment and prevention services. Combat stress is the emotional and physical stress experienced as a result of exposure to the inherent dangers and demand of serving in a combat environment. Combat operational stress reactions are expected, predictable intellectual, physical, emotional, and/or behavioral reactions of service members who have been exposed to stressful events in combat or in military operations other than war.[28] The COSC team's goal is to identify, prevent, and manage adverse and operational stress reactions.[29] COSC units provide education and therapy in the combat theater. They emphasize easy access to care and prevention. A primary goal of COSC is to reduce the stigma often associated with seeking mental health services.[30]

COSC dogs were assigned to work with occupational therapists. Occupational therapy is the use of everyday activities with individuals and groups for the purpose of participation in roles and situations at home, school, the workplace, the community, and other settings. Occupational therapy is provided for rehabilitation, and the promotion of health and wellness to those who have or are at risk for developing an illness, disease, condition, disorder, impairment, or limitation.[31] Occupational therapists provide direct patient care, readiness training, wellness education, and injury prevention to soldiers.[32]

Behavioral health programs are a primary mission for U.S. Army occupational therapists during combat operations.[33] In COSC, occupational therapists assess the service member's functional performance in daily living operations and work to prevent behavioral health casualties.[34] They provide education and therapy in the war theater and attempt to promote access to care and reduction of the stigma associated with seeking behavioral health care.[35] They work to develop positive relationships with neighboring units and commanders so that in times of need COSC staff will be trusted.

The COSC dogs worked as part of a program of prevention. Preventive mental health programs target not just those who are already stressed and suffering but those who might be at risk. Stress or the need for mental health services may be invisible and challenging to identify. Often, the person experiencing the symptoms needs to self-identify and seek out help. However, seeking help is often difficult due to the stigma associated with asking for assistance. At the same time, it is helpful to get preventive mental health services to those who can benefit from them as early as possible, even before symptoms develop. Early intervention and prevention involve encouraging people to see counselors and address any concerns proactively before deploying to combat zones or before symptoms develop.

Battling Stigma

A crucial part of Boe's and Budge's role was to help break down the stigma of talking with a mental health professional. Stigma occurs when one person or group has a negative view of another. This may happen because the person has a distinguishing personality characteristic or a trait that is or is thought to be a disadvantage (a negative stereotype). Negative attitudes and beliefs toward people who have a mental health problem are common.[36]

Many people in the general population who need mental health treatment do not seek it due to the stigma associated with mental illness.[37] Nearly two-thirds of all people with diagnosable mental disorders do not seek treatment.[38] They do not feel comfortable talking about their mental health issues and often internalize the stigma that is attached to them. This internalization can damage the hope for recovery.[39] An individual may begin to believe negative thoughts expressed by others about mental illness and the need for mental health assistance and think of themselves as hopeless and unable to recover. This may lead to shame, low self-esteem, and inability to achieve goals. Mental health conditions may worsen because the persons needing services do not receive the support and care they need to recover. Some people, to avoid being labeled mentally ill, refuse to seek care.[40] Mental illness can have a long-term impact on people's education, employment, physical health, and relationships. Stigma and negative attitudes within the military about obtaining mental health treatment often prevent those in need of care from receiving it.[41]

In 1999, a U.S. Surgeon General Report on Mental Health[42] identified stigma as a public health concern that leads people to "avoid living, socializing, working with, renting to, or employing individuals with mental illness." Mental illness and mental health concerns continue to be discussed in whispers and with shame.[43] The surgeon general's report recommended fresh approaches for researching stigma and developing measures to counter it.[44]

Many in need of mental health services, including military personnel, do not talk about their mental health problems.[45] In 2015, the RAND Corporation completed a study on mental health stigma in the military.[46] This study hypothesized that mental health stigma may be a barrier to mental health care seeking by the military and that these mental health symptoms can have a negative impact on the quality of life and social and cognitive function of military personnel. RAND researchers defined stigma as a "dynamic process by which a service member perceives or internalizes this brand or marked identity about himself or herself or people with mental health disorders."[47] This process occurs through the interaction between a service member and the community in which the service member resides. The report went on to identify stigma reduction strategies that seemed most promising and noted that stigma reduction requires a variety of innovative approaches, including the education of key groups about stigma, policies to reduce the stigmatizing behavior, and new stigma reduction programs.[48]

Using therapy dogs as social lubricants to reduce stigma is an example of an innovative approach to encourage early prevention for service members who have not yet developed symptoms of mental illness, thus decreasing stigma and encouraging early prevention and intervention.

Learning and Challenges

The new COSC therapy dog program resulted in both challenges and learning. One challenge was determining the optimal length of stay in the field for the COSC dogs. The first dogs, Boe and Budge, had two deployments totaling 24 months, which gave them ample experience in the field and established a baseline for researching the impact of such service on an individual dog. In 2009, Specialists Zeke and Albert were trained to replace Boe and Budge, and Boe and Budge returned to VetDogs, where they were reevaluated and retrained for service at Eisenhower Medical Center.[49] It then became standard procedure for America's VetDogs to meet a returning COSC unit and transport the dog back to Smithtown, where it was determined whether they should be redeployed or assigned to another mission.[50]

Other challenges were encountered in the first deployments of Boe and Budge.[51] Soldiers tended to give the dogs treats and snacks, and the dog's diet and fitness program needed to be modified. The therapy dog needed to be isolated from other feral animals. Well-intentioned persons would bring other dogs that were not trained or appropriately screened into therapy roles.[52] Another challenge for the new program was determining appropriate outcome measures and a way to measure program effectiveness.

Legacy

In 2010, two more dogs, Specialists Apollo and Timmy, were trained in Germany to accompany the 254th Medical Detachment to Afghanistan stationed at Bagram Airfield. In 2011, Zeke and Albert were reevaluated and reassigned to Eisenhower Medical Center. Albert remained at Eisenhower and Zeke redeployed to Afghanistan.[53] Between 2007 and 2011, a total of eight therapy dogs were deployed to Iraq and Afghanistan: Boe, Budge, Timmy, Zeke, Albert, Butch, Zach, and Apollo.[54] Most of the COSC dogs were reassigned to occupational therapy or physical therapy units at U.S. bases. Boe was assigned to Fort Benning, Georgia. Sergeant Budge died of lymphoma in July 2010, and had served two tours in Iraq, one each at Fort Hood and Fort Bragg, and a final assignment at Fort Gordon.[55]

The official COSC dog program stopped with the drawdown of troops. Since then, programs of animal-assisted intervention have become more numerous across the Department of Defense as the benefits of animal-assisted intervention have been demonstrated. Therapy dogs have been utilized in numerous programs, including unstructured wellness visits, visits of volunteer teams on hospital wards, and goal-oriented animal-assisted therapy in behavioral health clinics. Policy has been developed to address the use of therapy dogs in military treatment facilities.[56]

Jax, a German shepherd, joined the 163rd Attack Wing as a therapy dog and made visits to airmen in their work centers. Jax, who formerly trained as a police dog, served as a bridge between Director of Psychological Health David Cunningham and the unit. In 2016, Zoe, a Labrador retriever, joined the National Guard's 102nd intelligence wing. TOML (named for the pararescue motto "That Others May Live"), a year-old Labrador, joined the Alaska National Guard 212th rescue squadron and performed a variety of tasks to support the unit's mission and its personnel. In 2017, Ted, a German shepherd coonhound mix, joined the Wisconsin National Guard to interact with children before the unit's deployment. Apollo, a Labrador retriever from a local shelter, assisted the Sexual Assault Prevention and Response Office at White- man Air Force Base in Missouri. Lexy, a German Shepherd therapy dog, served with her partner, psychiatrist Major Rumayor at Fort Bragg.[57] Evolving trends in the military use of therapy dogs include expanded use of dogs for wounded soldiers and other service members and veterans, the use of dogs in overseas combat areas to assist with COSC, and the use of therapy dogs to help with post-traumatic stress disorder and other behavioral health concerns.[58]

In 2017, Rumayor and Thrasher[59] reviewed recent literature on animal- assisted therapy in the military and concluded that current research supports the structured use of therapy dogs in the treatment of specific conditions and with specific populations, although the need for studies with more rigorous methodology persists.

One area that has not been systematically studied is the effect of the service on the dogs. Rumayor and Thrasher noted that trends in the research call for increased consideration for the study of animal welfare. While studies have increased on how dogs help humans' mental and physical health, few studies have examined how serving in these assistance roles affects dogs. Dogs, like their human comrades, are impacted by war. The violence, trauma, chaos, and emotion affect them. As with humans, each dog's reaction is dif- ferent, and we still have much to learn about the effects.

The eight dogs who served in the first COSC dog program pioneered new roles in mental health and other supportive services for military per- sonnel. As more is learned more from the evolving science and study of animal-assisted interventions, especially for mental health programs, it will be interesting to see how the longstanding partnership between the military dog and the soldier will further evolve into invaluable mental health roles. The soldier-therapy dog team is likely to continue to inspire us by the loyalty, courage, and service of both human and canine soldiers and their example of health care innovation through human-canine collaboration.

8

A New Generation
of Therapy Dogs

Bevo, a 9-year-old yellow Labrador retriever, sits in a circle of 15 other dogs inside a church meeting room in Garland, Texas. Sunday is meeting day for the therapy dogs and their handlers. They are part of the Pet Partners of Greater Dallas, a community-based partner of the national Pet Partners therapy animal organization. Further down the line of chairs from Bevo, a line of 15 more dogs sit at attention at the feet of their handlers. The dogs are assorted sizes, ages, and breeds: a golden retriever, a Chihuahua, a Newfoundland, a Jack Russell terrier, and almost a dozen other dogs of assorted lineage. A few of the miniature breed dogs lounge in fleece-lined baskets held in their handler's lap. Most of the dogs, like Bevo, wear official therapy dog vests.

At the other end of the leash, handlers wearing yellow, white, and brown therapy dog t-shirts with the Pet Partners therapy dog insignia are taking notes. The human group is as diverse as the dogs—a mix of men and women of assorted ages and backgrounds. They are teachers, health care professionals, therapists, dog advocates, and retirees. Today they have a common identity. They are the human end of a therapy dog team.

Sitting on the floor alongside each handler-dog team is a knapsack embroidered with the dog's name and filled with the tools of the therapy dog's daily work. The teams carry the dog's calling cards, which look like baseball cards and feature the therapy dog's photo, resume and motto, and list of the dog's favorite hobbies. When the teams visit hospitals, nursing homes, schools, libraries, universities during exam weeks, and community events, the dog's calling cards are given to those they visit. Many children and adult fans of the dogs collect the dogs' cards, making sure they get one for each therapy dog they see. The cards are a big hit with the dogs' fans—and these days there are more and more fans. Today there are not enough therapy dogs to visit everyone who requests them. Demand for therapy dogs has exceeded supply since the Dallas group was organized in 2009.

Bevo's handler, Susan Schultz, is a co-founder and coordinator of the group, along with Carolyn Marr, another co-founder. Schultz is a retired licensed marriage and family counselor. She started the group with Marr, a director of rehabilitation, with Marr's registered therapy dog, Dolly, a long-coated Chihuahua. Schultz, Marr, and their dogs, Bevo and Dolly, are today's pioneers on the forefront of animal-assisted interventions (AAIs.) They witnessed firsthand the growth that has occurred in therapy animal work in the past decade. Schultz and Marr have been at it from the days when a dog was rarely seen in a hospital. Susan Schultz is a Pet Partners instructor, and Carolyn Marr is a Pet Partners evaluator.

Pet Partners of Greater Dallas is a community group of the national Pet Partners therapy animal organization, which was founded in 1977 as the Delta Society. Pet Partners connects people with the healing power of animals by providing volunteers and education and making therapy animal visits.[1] Pet Partners of Greater Dallas trains human volunteers and evaluates human-animal teams for participation in visiting therapy animal programs in local hospitals, nursing homes, rehabilitation centers, and schools. Training for volunteers is provided through hands-on and online workshops taught by Pet Partners–licensed instructors. Volunteers and their pets are then evaluated for skills and aptitude by Pet Partners licensed team evaluators such as Marr.

Schultz calls the meeting of dogs and handlers to order. She puts her partner, Bevo, in a down position, and he immediately complies. An occasional bark punctuates the discussion. A young golden retriever arrives late and interrupts the meeting as he barks a greeting to announce his arrival. The young golden immediately offers a perfect sit on the command of his handler. He is learning to be a registered therapy dog, and he is attending the meeting to learn proper meeting etiquette. Attending the monthly meeting with their handlers is part of the dogs' ongoing socialization process. The more experienced therapy dogs model the proper meeting behavior for the novices and mentor the rookies as they prepare to take the therapy dog evaluation to gain the registered therapy dog credential.

As dogs and humans settle, every canine and human head looks up to listen to instructions from Schultz who distributes handouts, and she makes rounds to each handler-therapy dog team. Bevo's tail wags faster as Schultz draws closer. Bevo knows that with the handout comes a gentle pat on the head.

As the monthly meeting of Pet Partners of Greater Dallas ends, new agency assignments and volunteer teams are matched, and dogs and handlers gather belongings, leashes, and knapsacks and get ready to adjourn. Everyone is looking forward to networking and catching up on the latest team news, but no one anticipates the adjournment more than Bevo and his fellow therapy dogs, who know that a few treats await them at the door. Before they leave, Schultz stops to remind them one more time: "We need more therapy dog teams."

Today, walk down the corridors of a hospital, and you might just meet friendly therapy dogs like Bevo and Dolly and their human handlers visiting with patients, families, and staff. The canine volunteers and their therapy dog colleagues are part of a new generation of registered therapy dogs and who have gained increased acceptance as an integrated part of the modern health care team. The journey required learning what dogs could teach us.

In the 1970s, Carolyn Marr was working in the mental health field with psychiatric patients who had been hospitalized for many years. Most had no family and rarely if ever left the hospital. Marr suspected these patients might not have touched an animal in years. A lifelong animal lover, she presented the idea of bringing animals into the hospital to visit patients, but the new approach was not initially well received.

Marr was determined. As a start, she developed policies to guide a small pilot project for animal visitation at the hospital. She was eventually successful and was permitted to begin a small animal visiting program with guinea pigs. This program was successful and popular with both staff and patients. Encouraged by the positive response to the small project, Marr worked to further develop an animal-assisted therapy (AAT) program. By the early 1990s, AAT was being offered hospital-wide.

By 2000, Marr was the director of rehabilitation at the large state psychiatric hospital. At this point, Marr and her colleagues had learned and understood that the key to developing and implementing animal-assisted programs in health care is research and data to support the evidence of its effectiveness. She and her colleagues studied the effects of AAT among their psychiatric patients and whether the interventions increased appropriate social behaviors. The study results suggested that patients who experienced AAT displayed more prosocial behaviors and were more interactive and participatory in their treatment program. Marr and her colleagues recommended more long-term studies of the effect of AAT.[2]

The AAT program developed by Marr and her colleagues evolved and grew with time over 25 years. In 2018, reflecting on the experience, Marr noted:

> It seems natural that based on the wonderful attributes that animals possess, such as unconditional love and the ability to discern emotional needs of humans, we would come to the realization that just as they have been our partners in our families, they could also be partners in comfort and healing for others.[3]

In 2008, Susan Schultz, a licensed marriage and family therapist, was beginning her journey into AAI work with Bevo, a 1-year-old yellow Labrador retriever. Bevo was a stray dog who had been adopted by Schultz and her husband. Schultz had been a puppy raiser for guide dogs and had a longstanding interest in mental health and animals. Schultz met Marr when Bevo was training to be a therapy dog. Marr was a Delta Society therapy animal evaluator. The two began collaboration and started to coordinate their therapy dog work.

As they mentored newly credentialed therapy dog teams, Schultz and Marr realized that the new therapy dog teams often struggled to find places and opportunities to visit with their dogs. They identified a need for therapy dog handlers to have a local learning network and a knowledge community to guide and evolve their common work. In 2009, Schultz and Marr brought together seven people with their idea to form a networking and support group for newly registered therapy animal teams and for those interested in working with therapy animals. The group adopted the name A New Leash on Life Therapy Animals of North Texas and began with members with therapy animals registered with the Delta Society. The Delta Society later changed its name to Pet Partners, and in 2017 the Dallas area group's name became Pet Partners of Greater Dallas.

The new Dallas area group gradually added more registered therapy dog teams. The founding members then approached area health facilities to inquire if they would like to have therapy dog teams visit their patients and clients. As the evidence and interest in AAT increased in the health community, opportunities to volunteer with therapy dogs increased.

By 2017, Pet Partners of Greater Dallas, which had started with just seven founding members, had a membership of over 100 volunteer animal therapy teams that provided close to 4,000 hours of animal-assisted activity a year to hospitals, assisted living facilities, nursing homes, and school reading programs throughout North Texas.[4] Today, Pet Partners of Greater Dallas is still adding teams of therapy dogs and their human partners but stretches its capacity to meet the increasing requests for therapy dogs for health care visits. Therapy dog teams from the group now visit most hospitals in the greater Dallas area. Each dog visits for a time limit of 2 hours. The therapy dogs walk the halls like rock stars and hand out their own calling cards to patients, families, and staff.[5]

Both Schultz and Marr credit the expansion in interest in AAT by health care facilities to an increased evidence base and a standards-based approach to their work. Both stress that hospitals and health care facilities want to know that teams and dogs are screened and qualified.[6] Marr said the biggest challenge in AAT has been and continues to be to maintain AAT professionalism—which means strict requirements for selection of handlers and animals based on the standards set by the national organization. A Pet Partners therapy animal team must qualify every two years.[7] Animals selected for therapy work are tested for temperament, evaluated for suitability for the work, and prepared.[8]

The Little Lady and the Labrador

Marr's dog Dolly was the first registered therapy dog in the new therapy dog networking group. A white, long-coated Chihuahua, the tiny canine made her therapy visits riding in a decorated basket labeled "chariot." Her diminutive size appealed to some adults and children who were not as comfortable with larger dogs. Dolly served as a small but mighty "diva and mentor" to the entire therapy dog group. A slow, low soft growl might emerge from the chariot when she felt the need to let the larger dogs know who had senior status. Dolly's calm demeanor, steady behavior, charisma, and willingness to socialize with people made her a perfect pioneer.

The tiny Chihuahua became a popular community ambassador. In addition to her pioneering work in health care facilities, Dolly was an ambassador for the role of therapy dogs to the local community. Dolly began to attend church with Marr. Sitting well behaved and attentive in her basket chariot next to Carolyn Marr each Sunday, Dolly became an "ambassadog" for therapy animals. Spurred on by Dolly's example of proper canine behavior in the pews, when the therapy dog group added more therapy dogs to their ranks, the church pastor and church congregation invited all the therapy dogs to attend services on Sunday. The therapy dogs of Pet Partners of Greater Dallas now have their own reserved pews and occasionally bark an amen or two to punctuate the pastor's remarks. Marr recalled seeing a slide one Sunday at a church presentation that read, "We give thanks for Dolly, who taught a congregation about wonderful programs and invited her friends."[9]

The church developed a tradition of celebrating the awarding of new credentials to therapy dogs with a commissioning ceremony. The first commissioning ceremony honored Dolly and Carolyn Marr as a registered Pet Partner team. Now when other newly credentialed therapy dogs have passed their qualifying test, they are invited to come to the communion rail to receive a commemorative bandana and a blessing to go out on their mission of service and caring. Each dog's photo and profile is flashed on the big screen as he or she is commissioned. The church now sponsors vaccination clinics, pet adoption events, a fundraiser for animal rescue, and an annual blessing of the animals.[10]

Marr recalled one of her most memorable experiences in therapy dog work. Dolly elicited an example of compassion and consideration unexpectedly when a young man came to read with Dolly. During a scheduled reading session, Marr asked the young man to select a book. The young man replied that he would like to read a particular one but he "didn't want to offend Dolly." The book was *The Old Dog*. Marr replied that she did not think Dolly would be offended at all. He read the first two pages and showed the pictures to Dolly. However, he kept putting his fingers on the next pages in a strange way. Marr was curious and asked about it. He said he was covering the word "old "so Dolly wouldn't see the word when he showed her the pictures. Said Marr, "That was a true 'heart tug' moment for me and was all about why I do what I do."[11]

Bevo, Schultz's muscular golden Labrador retriever, was Dolly's partner in pioneering the new therapy dog group. After completing his basic training and passing his qualifying exam, Bevo joined Dolly as a second dog pioneer of Pet Partners of Greater Dallas. Soon other new therapy dogs joined Bevo and Dolly as charter members of the new group. Bevo gained a reputation as somewhat of a prodigy since he had passed his therapy dog test the first time at just 1 year old, which is unusual for a such a young, frisky lab. Having passed his therapy dog test, Bevo went to work under Dolly's tutelage. Together Bevo and Dolly introduced the role of a therapy dog at facilities that had not previously had therapy dogs.

Bevo and Dolly both went on to earn credentials as reading education assistance dogs and visited libraries, schools, and health care facilities. Dolly and Bevo developed a close working relationship and social structure; Dolly made it clear that she might not surpass Bevo in weight and size, but she had seniority and authority. The combination of the large yellow muscular Lab and the petite, well-mannered Dolly in a basket made an irresistible combination when the duo appeared at the door to visit or read a story with a child. The Little Lady in the Basket and the Big Yellow Labrador led the way as more therapy dogs and their human partners joined the group.

A human-therapy dog team is a true partnership and a strong and enduring attachment. After a long career as Marr's therapy partner, Dolly at age 9½ died unexpectedly in 2015. The death hit her human partner hard. Marr admitted that it "took me a while to get my bearings." However, Dolly continued to show how a therapy dog impacts lives. Marr observed the overwhelming response to Dolly's death. She received flowers, cards, memory gifts, and even a beautiful plaque that now hangs in the church acknowledging Dolly's work. Marr remembered, "When I saw the love and tears for Dolly, I realized just how many lives she had touched, how instrumental she had been in helping to promote and advance animal-assisted activities and therapy—a true pioneer—a small four-pound lady who exemplified everything good about AAT and lived her life to show it."[12]

Today, Carolyn Marr continues her work as a therapy dog evaluator. She now makes her therapy dog visits with a new partner, Gabby, a tiny, white mixed Pekinese. Gabby carries on Dolly's tradition by visiting in a basket.

Bevo is still active in therapy work and makes therapy visits. Bevo is now a ranking senior leader in Pet Partners of Greater Dallas. Mature, fit, trim, and active, he keeps in shape on the treadmill and mentors new therapy dogs. Like all lifelong learners, Bevo receives continuing education to brush up on his skills. With over 200 therapy dog visits, Bevo has earned the American Kennel Club recognition title of both Excellent and Advanced. To receive this therapy dog recognition, a dog must be registered or certified by an American Kennel Club–recognized therapy dog organization and perform the number of visits for the title level for which they are applying. To receive the "Advanced" level, a team must have completed 100 visits; for "Excellent," 200 visits.[13]

Today, Pet Partners of Greater Dallas stretches its capacity to meet the number of requests for therapy animals to make health care visits. The demand for therapy dogs in health care facilities exceeds the supply of volunteer teams available.

The Trajectory of Animal-Assisted Interventions in Health Care

Slowly, as documented studies emerged, health care professionals became more interested in the impact of the human-animal bond and AAI. Physicians, health professionals, and the public were beginning to see the connection between the human-animal bond and human health.

Boris Levinson predicted that AAT would not be accepted without an increase in the documented evidence basis for its practice. Although the demand for therapy dogs in health care in modern health care facilities increased, true to Levinson's prediction, progress in developing such an evidence base for AAI was slow.[14]

Interest in the health benefits of pets and human-animal interactions increased after a 1987 workshop conducted by the National Institutes of Health focused on the health benefit of pets. This focus provided a catalyst to the quest for scientific research in animal-assisted interactions.[15] Interest in AAT from the general public began growing in the late 1990s and early 2000s. Several health care journals published articles documenting the benefits of AAT in a variety of health care settings.[16] The American Veterinary Medical Association initiated a Human-Animal Bond Task Force, and in 2006 a group of international representatives formed the International Society for Animal-Assisted Therapy with a focus on quality control, professional recognition, and continuing education in AAT.[17]

The four-decade history of the therapy animal organization Pet Partners illustrates the trajectory of AAI into mainstream health care. In the mid–1970s, a group of pioneers and volunteers—veterinarian Dr. Leo Bustad; psychiatrist Dr. Michael A. McCullough and his brother, Dr. William McCullough; and veterinarians Drs. R. K. Anderson, Stanley Diesch, and Alton Hopkin—

formed The Delta Foundation in Portland, Oregon. In 1981, the name was changed to the Delta Society.

Several key milestones highlighted the trajectory of the development of Pet Partners. In the early 1970s, the team of the McCulloughs published and supported Levinson's plea for more research, and Bill McCullough arranged for brother Michael to speak at engagements across the country. At that time, the press was skeptical and in writing about AAI, and the McCullough team was met with headlines such as "Psychiatrist goes to the dogs." The sentiment at the time seemed to be that the human-animal bond was just a passing fad for animal lovers.[18]

During this period the Delta concept evolved. The Delta triangle represented the client, the animal, and the veterinarian and recommended studying each of these sides of the triangle. The Delta Foundation was founded in Portland, Oregon, in 1977. The foundation later evolved into the Delta Society in 1983 with Dr. Leo Bustad as president. In the late 1980s, the Delta Society began to develop registration programs for AAT teams of therapy animals and handlers. In 2012, the Delta Society formally changed its name to Pet Partners and focused on providing direct animal-assisted services at the community level.[19]

The early board of directors was interdisciplinary and included veterinarians, a nurse, an MD, a social worker, a researcher, and a philanthropist. Another later milestone was the initiation of the American Veterinary Association, Task Force to study the profession's role in human-animal interactions. The first peer-review Delta Society Journal, *Anthrozoos*, was also established. The International Society of Anthrozoology (ISAZ) spun off to become a stand-alone organization and the largest publisher of Human-Animal Interaction research.

The Pet Partners Therapy Animal program was established in 1971, and Ann Howie and her dog Falstaff were the first registered pet partners in the nation. Pet Partners co-founded the international Association of Humane Animal Interactions Organization (IAHAIO).Standards of practice were established for AAT and AAA for health care facilities. The therapy animal continues to grow, improve, and evolve and a reading program "Read with Me" was established in 2018 to advance literacy.

In 2017, Dr. David Williams, the chief medical officer for Pet Partners, commented in *Pet Partners Interactions* magazine[20] on the trajectory of AAT in health care from the medical perspective. Williams noted that interest in AAI began over 200 years ago with Florence Nightingale's use of pets to reduce patient anxiety and Levinson's and Freud's use of dogs in psychotherapy. Dr. Williams noted that 40 years ago, most hospitals considered a dog's presence in a hospital as problematic for cleanliness and safety, but perception began to change when the Delta Society worked to ensure that animals and their handlers were educated, evaluated, and registered; more research demonstrated the health benefits of AAI; and patients provided feedback about the positive impact of therapy dog visits.[21] By 2016, Pet Partners reported that over 15,000 teams in all 50 states made 3 million visits.[22]

In addition to Pet Partners, several other national organizations offer testing, education, registration, credentialing and support for volunteer therapy animal handlers and their therapy dogs. These organizations include Therapy Dogs International and Alliance of Therapy Dogs, who provide therapy dog teams in health care and other settings.[23]

National mental health organizations have formally recognized the field of AAT.[24] In 2008, the American Psychological Association recognized the field and formed a new section, Human-Animal Interaction: Research and Practice, within Division 17 on Counseling.[25] The section is "dedicated to professional and scholarly activities that advance the understanding of human-animal interactions as they relate to psychology. HAI addresses the role of the human-animal bond in empathy development, the ability to form and express attachments, reaction to grief and loss, the challenges of aging, and other developmental passages throughout the lifespan." It also addresses "ways in which human interaction with animals promotes health" and "the role of animal-assisted therapies in prevention and intervention programs in a variety of settings."[26] The American Counseling Association Governing Council approved the establishment of the AAT in Mental Health Interest network in 2009.[27]

As AAI in health care has become recognized and more popular, a growing number of health care organizations in the United States and across the world have begun to implement animal-assisted programs. Increasing numbers of hospitals and health care organizations are interested in implementing facility animals or pet visitation to give patients the opportunity to interact safely with dogs and to make the hospital environment more comfortable and less stressful.[28]

Theories on the Human-Animal Bond

To understand what these modern therapy dogs do and can do in health care, it is helpful to know more about the human-animal bond. The human-canine interaction is a unique interspecies form of attachment. Observers have noticed for decades the positive effect animals can have on people's well-being. Early pioneer Florence Nightingale noted the beneficial effect of animals on the ill, and Freud and Levinson both noticed that their dogs Jofi and Jingles could facilitate psychotherapy.

In 2010, Kruger and Serpell wrote that the field of AAI currently lacked a unified, widely accepted, or empirically supported theoretical framework explaining how and why the human-animal bond is potentially helpful to human health.[29] No single theory has been adopted to explain the human-animal bond, but several mechanisms have been proposed to explain the positive effects of dogs on humans.[30] Kruger and Serpell then described various theories that have been used to explain how the human-animal bond works.[31] Theories related to attachment and social needs and the biophilia theory are particularly helpful in understanding the potential value of animals in therapeutic processes. AAI draws from these and other theories to describe the mechanisms for the therapeutic benefits of the human-animal bond.

The biophilia theory, introduced and popularized by Wilson in 1984, holds that human beings have an innate tendency to connect with other living things and are attracted by living organisms (animals). The biophilia hypothesis suggests that our natural affinity and attraction for nature and living things create our affinity for animals.[32]

According to social support theory, animals are a source of social support and companionship, which are necessary for well-being. The animal is part of our community and is an essential determinant of psychological well-being. Social mediation theorists hold that animals can serve as catalysts or mediators of social integration and can assist with rapport building between therapist and patient. Social support explains the close relationship people may form with animals.[33]

Theories of attachment emphasize the need for people to protect and be protected and people's tendency to attach to others. The theory describes social bonds that form with dogs as a further development of the most fundamental social bond—that between mother and child.[34] People's intense attachment to pets often mirrors human parent-child relationships. Attachment theory involves emotional bonds, seeking proximity and emotional and physical security and a functioning relationship between animals and humans.

Most of these mechanisms and theories as they relate to the human-animal bond have not been empirically tested, and this provides opportunities for future research in AAI.[35]

Trends in Research on Animal-Assisted Interventions

A gradual increase in the number of research studies to demonstrate the benefits of AAI propelled AAI forward as an adjunct modality in health care. A number of these studies presented results in various health care populations and, at the same time, described the need for more rigorous studies of AAI. Relatively few studies examined the effect of the work on the therapy dogs.

A common theme noted in a review of scientific literature about AAI is the need for more rigorous and well-designed studies. In 1984, veterinarian Alan Beck and psychiatrist Aaron Katcher published a review of studies on what was at the time termed pet-facilitated therapy.[36] They examined and analyzed existing studies and cautioned that only well-designed studies could demonstrate the effectiveness of animals as therapists. Beck and Katcher noted that Boris Levinson's case studies in pet-facilitated therapy were the best-known studies at the time and that "like any pioneer, he did not apply rigid experimental protocols but experimented with the flow of animals within the flow of therapy."[37] They also pointed out that there was no tabulation of Levinson's actual results. Beck and Katcher held that Levinson's work was unique in that no other psychologist had reported comparable experiences with animals, although many therapists worked with animals. They noted that anecdotal stories of the effectiveness of pet therapy did not prove the effectiveness and that the current evidence of the time lacked scientific rigor. Beck and Katcher explained that there are two types of studies: (1) descriptive studies that *generate* hypotheses or a research question, and (2) studies that *test* a hypothesis; all the current studies on pet-facilitated therapy were descriptive rather than hypothesis testing.[38] Descriptive studies are usually case studies, case results, or program reports. While evidence-based studies for AAT increased over the decades since Beck and Katcher published their review, their recommendation for more scientific study continues to be relevant today. In 2014, Borrego and colleagues also noted that progress in developing an empirical base for AAT had been slow and added that a gap remained between the research and its dissemination.[39]

Interest grew in the relationship between animals and human health, gradually increasing the body of evidence as research began to support the physical and psychological benefits of the human-animal bond.[40] More studies emerged to support the science behind AAT,[41] and several more recent reviews of AAI and AAT were conducted.[42]

Results from a 2015 meta-analysis[43] of AAT literature conducted by Nimer and Lundahl[44] supported the premise that animals can help in the healing process and that AAT is a robust intervention that deserves further use and study. Overall, AAT was associated with moderate effect sizes in improving outcomes in four areas: autism-spectrum symptoms, medical difficulties, behavioral problems, and emotional well-being. AAT showed promise as an additive to established interventions, and the authors suggested that future research should investigate the conditions under which AAT can be most helpful.[45] The data suggested that dogs have a greater chance of being effective than other animals, although the data could not answer why. Nimer and Lundahl's meta-analysis indicated that more research and theory development were still needed in AAT.

STUDIES OF AAI IN SPECIAL POPULATIONS

Studies of therapy dogs in action showed benefits in several health care populations. Cole and others studied adults hospitalized with advanced heart failure and found that patients who had a 12-minute visit with a volunteer and therapy dog had significant improvement in cardiopulmonary pressures, neurohormone levels, and anxiety compared with groups of patients who did not spend time with the therapy dog.[46]

AAI was found to benefit psychiatric patients. The animal-assisted activity helped decrease anxiety and increase socialization and social activity for hospitalized psychiatric patients. In 2014, Nepps and others found that patients hospitalized in a mental health facility who participated in a 1-hour animal-assisted activity session demonstrated significant decreases in depression, anxiety, and pain compared with another group that participated in stress management programs.[47] Barker and Dawson[48] found that AAT was associated with reduced anxiety levels for hospitalized patients with a variety of psychiatric diagnoses.

Research also demonstrated the link between human-animal interaction and healthy aging. One study found that AAT can effectively reduce loneliness in residents of long-term care facilities.[49] AAT has been shown to improve mood, psychosocial functioning, and quality of life in elderly dementia patients living in residential care facilities.[50] In a study of 68 nursing home residents in Australia, individuals who visited a dog reported less fatigue, tension, confusion, and depression.[51] Pet therapy was found to be effective in improving depressive symptoms and cognitive function in residents of long-term care facilities with mental illness.[52]

O'Haire and others concluded that AAI may provide promise as a complementary treatment option for trauma,[53] but noted that further research is essential to establish its feasibility and efficacy and to standardize protocols.

Researchers in a 2007 study found that patients receiving chemotherapy who received a visit by a therapy dog during the chemotherapy session had an improvement in depression and had higher oxygen saturation than the control group that did not have a therapy dog visit.[54] A study of children with cancer demonstrated that AAT plays a beneficial role in improving rest, nourishment, exercise, and socialization. AAT also played a role in lowering anxiety, overcoming problems, increasing motivation and self-esteem, and alleviating psychological distress in children and their parents. AAT facilitated coping with the therapeutic process and promoted the patient's well-being through-out hospitalization.[55]

In another study, AAT during counseling for breast cancer was successful in increasing patients' feelings of calmness, anticipation toward participating in counseling, the disclosure of information, and engagement with therapy while alleviating feelings of anxiety and promoting better communication with health professionals.[56] One study showed that cancer patients undergo-ing chemotherapy who had a weekly hour-long session of therapy with a dog rated their symptoms of depression and anxiety as half as severe as those who did not.[57]

Outside of the immediate health care environment, studies of therapy dogs interacting with college students at exam time found that students had reduced stress after AAI.[58]

Although a variety of AAIs have been introduced into health care to benefit patients and their families, the interventions have also been shown to have a positive effect on health care workers, who often have high levels of work-related stress. The inclusion of animals in the health care environ-ment has been shown to have a positive effect on staff members' stress levels and job satisfaction. Barker and colleagues noted that staff members volun-tarily played with therapy dogs that came to visit patients and observed that spending even short periods of time with the therapy dog could be effective in lowering staff members' cortisol levels.[59] Nurses also noted that observing a patient with a therapy dog enabled them to see a side of the patient's per-sonality that they wouldn't see otherwise, and this experience helped them better care for the "whole person."[60]

STUDIES OF AAI IN THE COMMUNITY

Even living with a companion animal has been shown to have beneficial effects. Today, 65 percent of U.S. households have pets; 69 percent of pet owners say that pets are important to their physical health, and 75 percent say that pets are important to their mental health.[61] Several studies have shown that people are happier and healthier in the presence of animals and have documented benefits of the human-animal bond, including reduced anxiety and enhanced feelings of well-being.[62] Positive human-animal interaction appears to be related to changes in physiological variables in both humans and animals, particularly dogs, including those variables associated with well-being.[63]

A 2018 study by Stull and colleagues in the *Journal of Gerontological Nursing* examined the frequency and types of animals in nursing homes and the perceived benefits of pet visits. The study also looked at the content of the organizations' policies addressing health risks. An online questionnaire revealed that animals were permitted in 99 percent of nursing homes. Dogs accounted for 95 percent of the visiting animals. Respondents perceived that animal interactions resulted in high health benefits for residents. Most respondents (75 percent) did not report health and safety concerns with animals in facilities. An interesting finding was that while most facilities reported having an animal policy, important gaps were identified in the content of policies. The researchers recommend that best practice guidelines and policies should be developed and implemented in nursing homes to address requirements for different animal ownership models, the range of animal species, and staff knowledge.[64]

WHAT ABOUT THE EFFECT OF AAI WORK ON THE DOGS?

While therapy dogs have been introduced in health care as adjuncts to therapy to promote human health and well-being, studies on the impact of the intervention on the animals themselves have been limited. In a review of available studies on therapy dog welfare during AAI, Glenk and colleagues[65] examined whether the integration of dogs in AAI promotes human well-being at the expense of animal well-being. The study concluded that the current body of evidence does not raise acute concerns for the welfare of dogs in the therapeutic environment, although more detailed study is needed into dogs' response to handlers' actions and the environment. An enhanced understanding of how dogs are influenced by environmental factors, AAI program features, and human handling may foster the promotion of successful teamwork and collaboration between humans and animals.[66]

In a study published in 2018 in *Applied Animal Behaviour Science*, Dr. Amy McCullough, a national director at the American Humane Association, with other researchers studied handler-dog therapy teams at five children's hospitals across the United States to determine the stress levels of dogs during regular AAI visits with pediatric oncology patients and their families.[67] A total of 26 therapy dog-handler teams were paired with newly diagnosed children with cancer. These teams provided regular AAI visits to the child and his/her parent(s) for four months. Canine saliva was collected at five baseline time points and 20 minutes after the start of study sessions for analysis of cortisol, a stress response hormone. The study team found that placing therapy dogs in a therapeutic setting did not increase their stress based on cortisol analysis as well as psychological and behavioral stress responses. The study called for more investigations on how therapy dogs deal with the demands of their work schedules on a long-term basis; in addition, a study of positive welfare indicators would determine if therapy dogs might actually benefit from their interactions in AAI.[68]

Guidelines to reduce work-related strain and to increase the quality of life of therapy animals have been published by the International Association of Human-Animal Interaction Organizations.[69]

FUTURE RESEARCH DIRECTIONS

Where are we now in the search for a sound research basis for AAI in health care? The lack of rigorous research is still a widely expressed critique of the field of AAI.[70] Methodological issues raised with existing studies have been small sample size, lack of control groups and random sampling, and lack of standardized protocols.[71] A frequent argument for more rigorous research is that many existing studies show correlation rather than causation. More studies are needed that demonstrate a cause-and-effect relationship between AAT and positive outcomes. For example, in a 2014 review of the literature of AAI in children's hospitals, Chur-Hansen and colleagues[72] noted that there was a perception in the scientific and general communities that hospitalized children benefit from visits by animals, yet the evidence base for the benefit was limited. Existing research studies in the area had methodological challenges that made conclusive statements about the efficacy of AAI difficult,[73] and therefore further research is still required.

While some of the evidence for AAI remains descriptive and anecdotal, scientific studies investigating the therapeutic effects of animals on human health are evolving into an organized collection of studies on the science of the human-animal bond and AAT. The Human-Animal Bond Research Institute (HABRI)[74] at Purdue University now houses, classifies, and archives research and information on the science of the human-animal bond. It has a comprehensive online database for human-animal bond research with more than 27,000 entries. HABRI Central,[75] a repository of resources, includes material from the fields of veterinary medicine, nursing, psychology, sociology, law, policymaking, and philosophy.

The Search for Common Terminology

Despite the long history of anecdotal and scientific reports of the positive benefits of AAI, there has been a lack of standardized terminology to describe AAI and the dogs involved in it. Not everything a therapy animal does is therapy. Not every helping dog is a therapy dog. A therapy dog is not a service dog. No wonder things get confused.

What's in a name? Names provide identity and clarity of roles, scope, and functions. The lack of clarity and precision in naming what animals do in animal-assisted programs has created difficulty for health care staff in understanding and identifying the appropriate scope for each of these levels of activity. That confusion, in turn, has resulted in difficulty determining appropriate target outcomes for the various types of AAI. This lack of clarity in names also created confusion among the public regarding the privileges and roles of each group of dogs.

It is helpful here to again clarify terms and consider the questions: What is the difference between animal-assisted therapy (AAT), animal-assisted activity (AAA), and animal-assisted education (AAE)? Public and service providers often define a broad range of interventions as AAT. Many sources that discuss therapy animals lump several types of animal-assisted programs into one generic category and refer to all of them as AAT. In many contexts, AAT has become a catchall term for a variety of AAIs.

In reality, AAI includes four different types of things that animals do: visiting, education, activity, and therapy. Each has a different scope and definition, but all require core competencies. As this terminology evolved and changed, these terms had inconsistent interpretations, which sometimes resulted in a different or inaccurate understanding of an animal's role and privileges.

ROLE DEFINITIONS

As important as it was to define the differences, no universally accepted definition existed for each level of AAI. However, in 2014, the International Association of Human-Animal Interaction Organizations published a white paper on the numerous and varied terms used to describe AAI. Members of the task force were academics, veterinary medicine professionals, and practitioners from different countries with a background or knowledge of different dimensions of human-animal interaction. The task force's goal was to clarify and make recommendations for AAI terminology. The task force also described ethical practices for the well-being of animals working in AAI. The following definitions were published by the IAHAIO (and are reprinted with permission)[76]:

- Animal-Assisted Invervention (AAI) "is a goal-oriented and structured intervention that intentionally includes or incorporates animals in health, education, or human service (e.g., social work) for the purpose of therapeutic gains in humans."[77]
- Animal-Assisted Therapy (AAT) "is a goal oriented, planned and structured therapeutic intervention directed and/or delivered by therapeutic and related service professionals. Intervention progress is measured and included in the professional documentation. AAT is delivered and/or directed by a formally trained (with active licensure, degree or equivalent) professional with expertise within the scope of the professionals' practice."[78]

- Animal-Assisted Activity (AAA) "is a planned and goal-oriented informal interaction and visitation conducted by the human-animal team for motivational, educational and recreational purposes."[79]
- "Animal-Assisted Education (AAE) is a goal oriented, planned and structured intervention directed and/or delivered by educational and related service professional. AAE is conducted by a qualified (with a degree) general and special education teacher. Regular education teachers who conduct AAE must have knowledge of the animals involved."[80]

ANIMAL-ASSISTED THERAPY

AAT strategically incorporates human-animal interactions into a formal therapeutic process,[81] while animal-assisted activity involves social visits with an animal. AAT is practiced as an adjunct to existing therapy but is integrated into the treatment process. A therapist incorporates the animal interventions into whatever type of professional therapy he or she practices. For example, a physical therapist provides physical therapy facilitated by a therapy animal, whereas a psychotherapist provides psychotherapy facilitated by a therapy animal.

An example of AAT is therapy dogs' work in rehabilitation. In rehabilitation treatment, AAT goals might include improving motor skills, walking skills, or wheelchair skills and improving range of motion of extremities. The therapy dog helps the therapist motivate the patient by engaging in activities with the patient. The patient might be encouraged to groom the dog, throw a ball, or stroke the dog. A therapy dog might work with a patient who uses a wheelchair by riding in the patient's lap while the person wheels to a designated place on an obstacle course. A patient who is working on improving the quality of his or her gait might work with a dog doing basic obedience skill training with the dog, placing the dog at the station at a sit while walking to the animal. The AAT visit is goal-directed with a specific end in mind.[82] The human-animal interaction is utilized as an adjunct to therapy delivered by a licensed professional and enhances the benefits of the therapeutic process.

ANIMAL-ASSISTED ACTIVITY

In contrast to AAT, animal-assisted activity involves interaction that is more informal or visitations often conducted on a volunteer basis by the human-animal team for motivational, comfort, support, educational, and recreational purposes. Human-animal teams who provide animal-assisted activity may also work formally and directly with a health care provider, educator, and/or human service provider on specific, documentable goals. Animal-assisted activity in health care settings might occur at special events, at staff meetings, as well as room-to-room patient social visits. Animal-assisted activity also includes animal-assisted crisis response that focuses on providing comfort and support for trauma, crisis, and disaster survivors and visiting community.[83]

THERAPY DOGS VS. SERVICE DOGS

In exploring the role of therapy dogs, it is also helpful to review the differences between therapy and service dogs. A *therapy dog* visits with a handler to provide affection and comfort to various members of the public, typically in a variety of facility settings such as hospitals, retirement homes, and schools. Therapy dogs have no special rights of access, except in those facilities where they are welcomed. Therapy dog teams pass a test by a national organization that shows that the handler and animal are suitable. Therapy dog teams are volunteers, and the dogs are personal pets. They are used as part of a treatment program in AAT, or in less formal, social activity as an animal-assisted activity.[84]

An *assistance dog* is an animal supporting people who have disabilities. Assistance dogs are also commonly called *service dogs*. An assistance or service animal is a dog that has been individually trained to do work or perform tasks for an individual with a disability. A *guide dog* is a service dog who has been trained to assist a blind or visually impaired person.

Therapy dogs and service dogs have different rights of access. Assistance dogs are considered working animals, not pets. Assistance or service dogs are permitted, in accordance with the Americans with Disabilities Act, to accompany a person with a disability almost anywhere the public is allowed.[85]

A *facility dog* is an animal who is regularly present in a residential or clinical setting. The dog might live with a handler who is an employee of the facility and come to work each day or might live at the facility full time under the care of a primary staff person. Facility animals should be specially trained for extended interactions with clients or residents of the facility, which may include animal-assisted activity, AAE, or AAT.[86]

The Therapy Dog at Work: Both Art and Science

No one knows how to work a room like a therapy dog. Anyone who has observed a therapy dog in action soon realizes there is an art, as well as a science, to what a therapy dog does. Bellin, a majestic rescued husky in Texas with a powerful message, demonstrates this art and poetry of the therapy dog as he shows and tells his own story of healing, hope and his example of resilience.

BELLIN BELLIN: "IF I CAN, YOU CAN TOO"

In 2011, pediatrician Kassia Kubena-Fontenot and her husband Steve were volunteers for Texas Husky Rescue when San Antonio Animal Care Services called them about an abused husky. The husky had repeatedly been beaten, was weak and lethargic, and had been left without shelter, food, and water for days. The Fontenots fostered the traumatized husky and then adopted him in January 2012. They named the husky Bellin Bellin for a wind god who blew the winds of change. The name would prove to be prophetic for the journey the three would travel together. At first, Bellin would not even acknowledge his new human family. The dog just slept, ate, and went outside when needed. Yet, somehow, he seemed to know he was safe and he began healing in body and spirit. Bellin became curious about his new world. He showed an exceptional ability to connect with people.

The Fontenots thought Bellin might be a good therapy dog, and all three started the journey to becoming a therapy team. In 2013, Bellin and Kassia were evaluated by Therapy Animals of San Antonio and registered as a Pet Partners team.[87]

Bellin Bellin works where his inspiring story of courage provides a message of hope and resilience. Bellin's first therapy visits were at Kubena Pediatrics, Dr. Fontenot's medical practice. "Team Bellin" then went on to visit the Children's Bereavement Center of South Texas, Methodist Children's Hospital San Antonio, oncology units, and the San Antonio Children's Shelter and other health care sites. At the Children's Bereavement Center, children often have a difficult time opening up about grief and loss. Bellin lies down next to them. The children play with his hair or just pet him. Before they know it, they will start to talk about emotions, and their grief about their lost loved one. Bellin and his story of recovery and resilience inspires those he meets who have their own challenges to overcome. His message is: "I am Bellin. If I can come back, you can too."[88]

In 2013, all three members of Team Bellin, Dr. Kubena-Fontenot, Steve Fontenot, and Bellin, began visiting in an adult oncology unit. The hospital and staff were thrilled to see how deeply the patients connected to Bellin and how he brought smiles and comfort to patients who were fighting for their lives. A few weeks later, Bellin made his debut at a children's hospital emergency department around Thanksgiving. Bellin's visit made a difference in the outlook of everyone—doctors, staff, and patients alike. The staff was laughing and having fun as they watched some of the kids forget they were sick and saw how the parents' worry was replaced with a smile. Steve Fontenot recalled: "We didn't know it [at] that time, but this would be the start of Bellin making holiday rounds. Since then, Bellin has visited the emergency department on almost every major holiday."[89] *It wasn't long until Bellin was part of the emergency room staff. Steve Fontenot observed:*

In the past decade, health care professionals have been opening up various alternative therapies including AAT. They are becoming more aware of the scientific studies showing a decrease in heart rate, blood pressure, and stress hormones like cortisol following AAT. Therapy animals don't just visit patients; they visit staff and families of patients. In a place like an emergency room or anywhere in the hospital where stress and anxiety run high, AAT can be just what the doctor ordered.[90]

In 2018, Bellin looked forward to retirement having completed almost 1,000 hours of visiting logged since he began his work as a therapy dog. He pioneered the role of the therapy dog expanding his work into new health care venues, touching those who most needed his message of hope and resilience.

In his foreword to Fine's *Handbook on Animal-Assisted Therapy*, Stanley Coren described the power of witnessing the connection between dog and patient.

> Actually observing the effects an animal can have in ameliorating a psychological problem sometimes has the emotional effect that might be expected if you observe something miraculous.[91]

The work of dogs like Bellin can truly seem miraculous. It's important to note, however, that the art of therapy dogs is not "magic"; the dogs do not possess special healing powers. Instead, as Risë VanFleet and Faa-Thompson explained in their book, *Animal Assisted Play Therapy*,[92] thinking of AAT as magical does not allow for defining the work or reproducing the results in clinical practice or study. Expecting an animal to magically sense what a human needs puts an undue responsibility on the animal. Animals are not the therapist; they assist the therapist. The animals act as a bridge between the client and the therapist, who applies principles and knowledge in his or her therapeutic practice.[93]

The art of the therapy dog is the human-animal collaboration and teamwork and the reciprocal relationship of the human and dog that emerges in the AAT session and allows the dog to facilitate the therapeutic techniques being provided by the licensed professional. It is the visible representation of the human-animal bond.

Each therapy dog finds his or her own niche. Not every therapy dog in a health care setting has the same purpose or role. Like humans, dogs are good at different things. As health care organizations integrate AAT into their programs for patients and staff, therapy dogs may work in several areas, including rehabilitation, counseling and psychotherapy, occupational and physical therapy, and social visiting in health care facilities. Therapy dog teams may informally visit with patients, families, or health care staff or provide goal-directed interventions under the direction of a licensed professional clinician such as an occupational therapist, physical therapist, social worker, or child life specialist.[94] Therapy dogs can also serve as symbols, social lubricants, sources of inspiration and comfort, and metaphors.

How can dogs do all this?

One of the things that make animals so unique in a hospital or health care environment is their ability to touch people, physically and psychologically.[95] Humans and dogs are social animals. We need each other. Humans and animals both need to be connected. Pets can nurture us and give us an opportunity to nurture. The presence of a therapy animal for a depressed patient or family gives them the chance to nurture that animal, a brief respite from being in the patient role. They may "give" to the animal the comfort or nurturing that they so badly need but have difficulty expressing to their own caregivers. As friendly animals convey a sense of social friendliness, there often is a healing presence. With a therapy dog visit, a patient may feel comfort, acceptance, or affection without judgment or expectation. This may be difficult for the person in pain or crisis in a busy hospital. A therapy dog can open the door to the expression of thoughts and feelings on the minds of patients or family members, and even hospital staff.

Engaging in play or caring for an animal can brighten a person's mood or affect, and he or she learns how to experience pleasure in the real moments of life. Just petting a dog is soothing and hearing a comforting dog story can be calming. With both children and adults, a storytelling session about an animal's history, with the animal present, provides an abundant opportunity both for creative narrative and for the added experiential impact of getting and receiving touch from the animal.

THERAPY DOGS IN COUNSELING AND PSYCHOTHERAPY

Just as Jofi and Jingles assisted Freud and Levinson, the modern therapy dog sometimes assists in counseling and psychotherapy. A therapy dog can help build an atmosphere of trust between a client and the therapist. Interventions with an animal can also improve social skills, brighten a patient's affect and mood, and improve memory and recall. The therapy dog intervention may also address grief/loss issues, improve cooperation, and enhance a patient's ability to trust.[96] Like Levinson's work with Jingles, the client and therapist might talk about the dog, introduce the dog to others, and give and receive affection from the dog. The client might tell the therapy dog or the therapist about animals he or she has known, observe the dog's reaction to other people or discuss how the therapy animal might feel.

A therapy dog sometimes helps someone to reveal or project his or her own concerns. A patient can begin to understand and tell his or her own story by talking about the therapy dog. An example is a patient worried while awaiting test results. (Let's use Jingles as an example here.) After a few visits with Levinson's dog, a young patient might remark, "I think Jingles looks worried about something today." In this type of interaction, a therapist might just remain silent and listen to what comes next or ask, "What do you think Jingles has on his mind?" or "What do you think Jingles feels about that?" Dr. Cynthia Chandler, writing in her book *Animal-Assisted Therapy in Counseling*, described this type of working with a therapy dog as a "side door technique" of having a client imagine what the animals experience.[97]

Therapy dogs may assist in counseling and psychotherapy with several other interventions, such as storytelling and the use of animal-assisted metaphors. O'Callaghan and Chandler have identified 18 different techniques and 10 intentions for AAT in mental health.[98]

In an animal-assisted metaphor, listeners shift their attention to the animal and interpret the story from their own perspective. In hearing or telling a story about an animal, individuals can relate to frightening or worrisome content because it is less threatening than the reality.[99] Animals are often symbols and can represent an adult's inner world. As an example, Florence Nightingale's first patient, the sheepdog Cap, may have become a symbol of her search for her life's healing purpose.

Outside of therapy environments, dogs participating in an animal-assisted activity or animal-assisted education touch lives in many different ways when they interact with people on a more social basis. A therapy dog can act as a kind of canine storyteller, speaking to us without words. Reading assistance dogs listen attentively as a child reads to them or we tell them our troubles and our story. They are nonjudgmental listeners who do not criticize a struggling reader or tell them what to do. Giving affection to an animal, or hearing a story about a dog like Bellin who triumphs over adversity to receive love and affection, may help reduce a person's feelings of hopelessness, boredom, isolation, and loneliness.

Therapy dogs serve as symbols, metaphors, inspiration, and comfort and nonjudgmental listeners. With a therapy animal present, a human has the comfort and communication of another living spirit. Dogs are often the first to hear our untold story—the story that we are afraid to tell anyone else.

From Pioneers to Professionals

How many organizations welcome therapy animals today? There is no standardized and systematic way to measure the number or determine specifics about the programs and their effectiveness.[100] There is also a lack of information about what areas or units of the hospital therapy dogs are allowed to visit, how many therapy dogs visit the hospitals, what dog breeds are permitted, how often visits occur and for how long, and what other species of animals are allowed to participate.[101]

While there is no current standard protocol for therapy dog programs in a hospital, most health care organizations have a program model with core policies and procedures. The basic model for AAT is similar, but the existing literature shows that there is "substantial variation in practice,"[102] such as the areas of an organization a therapy dog is allowed to visit.

While therapy animal visits to health care facilities can provide health benefits to individuals, they can also represent health risks.[103] Professionals involved in AAI must work to reduce the risk of clients and ensure that safety measures are in place.

QUALIFICATIONS FOR DOGS AND HANDLERS

Not every "pet in a vest" is a therapy dog. The dog must qualify and meet the criteria established by the credentialing therapy dog organization. Not every dog can be a therapy dog. It takes specific characteristics for a dog to make a good therapy dog. The human end of the leash also must possess certain characteristics.

Therapy animals must want to visit, be friendly and confident, know how to respect personal boundaries and be nonaggressive, controllable, predictable, and reliable. A potential candidate will initiate contact, stay engaged, make eye contact, and allow his or her behaviors to be redirected.[104]

Volunteer animal handler teams working in health care facilities are typically required to be trained and registered with a national therapy animal organization. When volunteering in a health care organization, handlers are required to complete hospital volunteer training and orientation, which discusses hospital policies such as confidentiality and privacy. Many organizations require the handler to complete health clearances.

ORGANIZATIONAL POLICIES

While more and more hospitals and health care facilities are bringing in therapy dogs, many have yet to develop policies and procedures to guide them.[105] An August 2017 study surveyed U.S. hospitals, eldercare facilities, and therapy animal programs to assess health and safety policies related to AAT. The study found gaps between the policies of facilities and current guidelines for animal visitation and indicated that programs need to review their policies to address recent guidelines.[106] There is a continuing need for common terminology, defined roles, and standards of practice, implementation guidelines, policies, and comparable measures of success.

Core requirements for a hospital animal-assisted visiting program or intervention program include the development of program goals, policies, procedures, organizational infrastructure and ownership, outcome and continuous improvement measures, and plans for integration and communication. Policies are needed for safety, regulatory guidelines, patient selection, handler requirements, credentialing, confidentiality, ethics, infection control, health screening for both animals and handlers, background checks for handlers, volunteer orientations, medical record documentation for AAT visits, communication with organizational caregivers, and actual patient interactions.[107] These elements are essential for advancing and integrating the promise of the human-animal bond into today's health care.

GUIDELINES AND BEST PRACTICES

Care of both human and animal members of the health care team requires guidelines and standards as AAI becomes integrated into health care settings. The International Association of Human-Animal Interaction Organizations (IAHAIO), in addition to publishing definitions for AAI, has published guidelines for human and animal well-being in AAI and best practices in AAI.[108] IAHAIO's revised White Paper on Definitions for Animal Assisted Intervention and Guidelines for Wellness of Animals Involved was first published in 2014 and updated in April 2018. The IAHAIO Guidelines stress that it would be unethical to initiate an AAI with a goal of improving a patient's welfare through a program that compromises the well-being of the animal or other individuals. In designing effective AAIs, facilities and handlers must ensure that adequate provisions and protocols are in place to continually monitor and safeguard the health and well-being of all patients, staff, handlers, visitors, and animals involved. Key IAHAIO recommendations include that handlers and professionals working with animals are trained and knowledgeable about the animals' well-being and are able to detect discomfort, distress, and stress. Professionals must have an understanding of normal animal boundaries and be respectful of them, and they should supervise clients at all times so that neither the client nor the animal is placed at risk.[109] Additional IAHAIO guidelines are that safety measures to reduce risks for clients must be in place. AAI should only be performed with the assistance of domestic animals that are in good health, both physically and emotionally, and that enjoy AAI activity. Professionals are held accountable for the well-being of the animals they are working with. Professionals must understand that the participating animal, independent of the species, is not simply a tool, but a living being. The IAHAIO best practices recommend that animals in AAI be registered with one of the national/international organizations as meeting certain criteria and indicate that not all animals, including many that would be considered "good pets" by their owners, are good candidates for AAI. Only domestic animals with the proper disposition and training should be selected for AAI. Regular evaluations should be performed to ensure that the animals continue to show proper disposition. A veterinarian should also examine animals considered for AAI before their involvement—assessing them for health and ensuring that all appropriate preventive medicine protocols are in place. For resident animals, veterinarians can also ensure that the environment and recipient group would suit their needs. Animals participating in AAI should never be involved in a way that would jeopardize their safety and comfort. The following are excerpts from the IAHAIO Guidelines for Human and Animal Wellbeing in AAI:

Human Well Being

- Safety measures for clients must be in place. Professionals must reduce risk for clients involved in AAI. They must ensure that clients do not have species or breed specific allergies, be aware of high risk in some population and of exclusion criteria depending on the risk (e.g., infection in immunosuppressed patients, and diseases which can be spread from client to client via the animal. In some situations, for example, working with immunosuppressed patients, public health specialists may require screening tests for animals to ensure they are not carrying particular infections).

- Animal handlers need to understand the needs of the recipients involved. They should have received training in the human context in which the AAI will occur.

- Recipients may have different views about specific animals included in interventions. When the recipients' beliefs—religious, cultural, or otherwise—run counter to recommended AAI, it is advisable that professionals discuss alternatives with recipients or their families, if incapacitated.

Animal Wellbeing

- AAI should only be performed with the assistance of animals that are in good health, both physically and emotionally and that enjoy this type of activity. It is mandatory that handlers must be familiar with the individual animals taking part in an intervention. Professionals are held accountable for the well-being of the animals they are working with. In all AAI, professionals need to consider the safety and welfare of all participants. Professionals must understand that the participating animal, independent of the species, is not simply a tool, but a living being.

- Only domesticated animals can be involved in interventions and activities. Domesticated animals (e.g., dogs, cats, horses, farm animals, guinea pigs, rats, fish, birds) are those animals that have been adapted for social interactions with humans. Domesticated animals must be well socialized with humans and trained with humane techniques, such as positive reinforcement. Domesticated animals (dogs, cats, equines) should be registered with one of the national/international organization as meeting certain criteria.

- Not all animals, including many that would be considered "good pets" by their owners, are good candidates for AAI. Animals considered for participation in AAI or AAA should be carefully evaluated for behavior and temperament by an expert in animal behavior such as veterinarians and animal behaviorists. Only those with the proper disposition and training should be selected for AAI. Regular evaluations should be performed to ensure that the animals continue to show proper disposition. A veterinarian should also examine animals considered for AAI before their involvement with recipients—assessing them for health, and ensuring that all appropriate preventive medicine protocols are in place, and for resident animals ensuring that the environment and recipient group would suit their needs.

- Handlers and professionals working with animals should have received training and knowledge of the animals' well-being needs, including being able to detect signs of discomfort and stress. Professionals should have taken a course on general animal behavior and appropriate human-animal interactions and species-specific (i.e., horses, pigs, hamsters, gerbils, and others) interactions.

- Professionals must have an understanding of animal specific boundaries that are normal and respectful to them. Animals participating in AAI should never be involved in such ways that their safety and comfort are jeopardized. Examples of such inappropriate activities and therapy exercises include, but are not limited to, recipients (children and adults) jumping or bending over animals, dressing up animals in human clothes or costumes, outfitting animals with uncomfortable accessories (dressing other than clothes such as bandanas, weather related jackets, booties designed specifically for animals), or asking an animal to perform physically challenging or stressful tasks (e.g., crawling, leaning/bending in unnatural positions). © IAHAIO 2014– 2018; used with permission.

In addition to the International Association of Human-Animal Interaction Organizations, several other organizations now provide guidance to health care organizations that seek to integrate AAT or animal-assisted activity into their programs. Infection control organizations have published recommendations related to animal-assisted programs in hospitals, which are now incorporated in program planning. The Society for Healthcare Epidemiology of

America outlined recommendations for the development of policies for AAT in health care facilities.[110] The guidance was also endorsed by the Association for Professionals in Infection Control and Epidemiology, a professional association of more than 15,000 infection prevention experts.[111] The American Association of Professionals in Infection Control and Epidemiology created guidelines that include hand hygiene, program management education, and visiting procedures.[112]

Beyond the infection guidelines, the American Veterinary Medical Association has established guidelines for animals participating in AAI and resident animal programs.[113] These guidelines address measures that should be taken to ensure the wellness of animals participating in AAI.

The Next Generation of Pioneers

Despite the growing body of evidence that animal assisted interventions can be helpful to human health, the full integration of animals into mainstream treatment methods may continue to move slowly until clinicians who prescribe treatments are convinced that therapy animals have therapeutic value. Not everyone agrees that the evidence is sufficient. The search for an evidence base for AAT continues by scholars and committed researchers and professionals of many disciplines. More rigorous studies are needed to better understand the cause-and-effect relationship as well as correlations and contributors to the effectiveness of the interventions.[114]

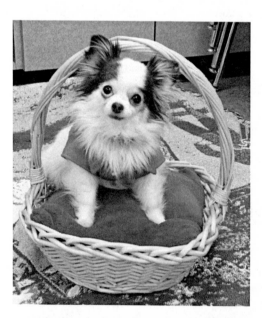

Today, animals serve as partners in animal-assisted programs. Animals are not "used" but instead intentionally integrated into the care system. AAI in health care settings requires a safe and beneficial environment for humans and animal partners, where they are viewed not as objects, but as living, breathing, and feeling members of a team.

Peter Rabinowitz, M.D., M.P.H., directs the Center for One

Dolly, a therapy dog pioneer, gets ready to visit in her "chariot," ca. 2015 (courtesy Carolyn Marr).

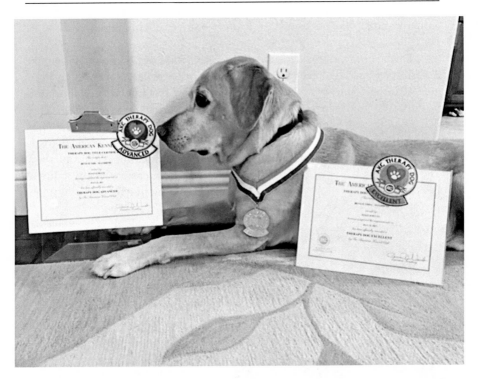

Bevo, a therapy dog pioneer, poses with his awards, ca. 2016 (courtesy Susan Schultz).

Health Research. The One Health project explores linkages between human, animal, and environmental health. Rabinowitz has described the role of health care professionals in human-animal bond issues, outlining essential competencies.[115] He has explained that the roles of health care providers may include acknowledger of the importance of the bond, prescriber of AAT, facilitator of AAI, certifier of support or assistance animals, and manager of animal-related health issues. As gatekeepers to health care settings, health care providers may be in a position to develop policies that facilitate AAT or other human-animal interactions.[116] Rabinowitz also noted that science, which continues to show the impact of the human-animal bond, may propel actions that support high-quality animal therapy programs in medical treatment and rehabilitation facilities. An essential first step is for health care providers to acknowledge the power of the human-animal bond, including its impact in medical situations, such as when a patient is hospitalized with a pet at home and when a pet dies. In spite of these roles, surprisingly, health care providers receive little or no education on the human-animal bond.[117] Additional curricula on the human-animal bond in health care providers' education can provide educated and informed health care leaders who advocate for incorporating animals into human health care in a safe, effective, and outcome-based manner.

The healing nature of animals in health care is both an art and a science. A variety of barriers have existed, but the most significant barrier has been lack of understanding and imagination of what interspecies collaboration can do. As a new generation of therapy dogs is integrated into health care delivery, they will show us still more about the art and science of AAI. They will create new paths in One Health, an initiative that unites human and veterinary medicine; teach us more about the effectiveness of AAT, and show us ways to increase the mutuality of the human-animal bond and interspecies collaboration.

As dogs and humans move forward together, dogs like Bevo, Dolly, Rusty, Bellin, and other modern therapy dogs will show us the impact of the human-animal bond in healing and human health. Dogs like Chi Chi, a golden retriever with four prosthetic legs who works as a therapy dog, will show us about overcoming handicaps and tragedy. Chi had been left for dead in South Korea in a garbage bag. The golden retriever's legs were tied up and eventually had to be amputated to save her life. Chi Chi was rescued and brought to the United States where she became a therapy dog. For her efforts inspiring others to face challenges in their own health and rehabilitation, Chi Chi was honored by the American Humane Association with their Hero Dog Award.[118] Our next generation of dog pioneers are waiting for their visionary human handlers to find them.

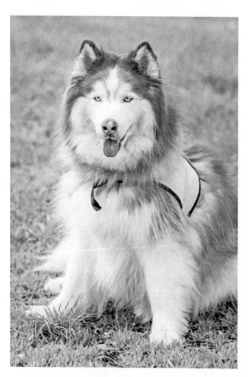

Bellin, a rescued husky and therapy dog, convinces people overcoming challenging circumstances, "If I can, you can too!," ca. 2018 (photograph by Raleigh Meade, courtesy Steve Fontenot).

9

Pioneers, Poetry and Possibilities

People who love animals, and who spend a lot of time with animals, often start to feel intuitively that there's more to animals than meets the eye. They just don't know what it is, or how to describe it.—Temple Grandin[1]

A surprising thing happened when humans began paying closer attention to dogs. As we watched our dogs work, we became curious about the science and poetry of the human-animal bond and the possibilities of interspecies collaboration in healing and health care. The Dog Pioneers helped health care providers imagine how interspecies collaboration might become part of health care innovation and improvement.

Health care is collaborative. It requires teamwork. Without health care providers' ability to work as a team, improvements and change are not possible. The Dog Pioneers of health care were the first to show humans how dogs could help us improve human health if we collaborated with them and invited them to join us on the health care team.

When we reflect on the stories of the Dog Pioneer, we can envision a future with our dogs at our side in health care delivery. Pioneers like the Mercy Dogs, Jofi, Jingles, the Serum Run sled dogs, Buddy, and the COSC dogs were leaders in interspecies collaboration. A simple sheepdog may have inspired Florence Nightingale's health care contribution. Dogs rushed to the side of the warrior on the battlefield, worked in the office of the psychotherapist, inspired the heroic narrative of Florence Nightingale, led medical supplies across the wilderness trails of Alaska, and navigated treacherous urban streets at the side of a blind person. These Dog Pioneers served as muse, inspiration, patriot, metaphor, and myth to inspire generations. They demonstrated the power of the symbolism of animals in healing narratives. Today, therapy Dog Pioneers continue to break into new roles in the world of modern medicine.

The Dog Pioneers' contributions spanned health care over many decades. *The Mercy Dogs* were trained to be first responders on the battlefield in World War I. They practiced the new art of triage and provided comfort to a soldier even as he lay dying on the battlefield. The Mercy Dogs were a symbol of patriotism and sacrifice.

As the storms of World War II gathered, *Jofi* was a pioneer in the developing science of psychoanalysis. Sigmund Freud studied his beloved chow to understand his patients. Freud and Jofi collaborated and introduced and validated the unheard-of concept of a canine co-therapist in the psychiatrist's consulting room.

Events with dogs can take on symbolic meaning, and symbols can evoke feelings and mobilize energy for change. *Cap*, an injured sheepdog, may have played a role in the trajectory of Florence Nightingale's life of health care reform. Although we only speculate on the depth and manner of Florence Nightingale's first patient's inspiration to her, we know that Nightingale's early experience with Cap became a part of Nightingale's heroic narrative of healing. She was a lifelong animal lover and an early proponent of animal-assisted intervention in health care. An encounter with the injured collie may have impacted her contributions to nursing, public health, health care reform, and health care statistics.

Balto, Togo, and the sled dogs of the serum run advanced public health in a diphtheria epidemic in the Alaska frontier. The two sled dogs were portrayed as heroes in newspapers across the United States, and their story is still used today to illustrate the importance of immunization. The dramatic transport of badly needed serum to Nome spurred development of more efficient air routes and better medical supply movement. The inoculation campaign dramatically reduced the threat of the disease.

Buddy, a German shepherd dog, crossed the Atlantic with Morris Frank as a pioneering guide dog for the blind. Together, Buddy and Morris Frank demonstrated that blind people were not helpless and that a human-animal partnership could bring new light and independence to the darkness of disability. Buddy established the working guide dog as a suitable partner for those who needed assistance. She inspired a new vision for those who were visually impaired and new access for assistance dogs in America.

In the 1960s, *Jingles* and psychologist Boris Levinson pioneered pet child psychotherapy, and Levinson's classic textbook *Pet-Oriented Child* Psychotherapy was inspired by their partnership. Although Levinson's colleagues initially ridiculed him for his ideas on the benefits of animals in psychotherapy, Levinson was inspired by Jingles to continue his pioneering work and to write on animal-assisted therapy. Levinson's book on pet-oriented psychotherapy still stands as a breakthrough reference in animal-assisted child therapy, and therapy dogs today work with young patients to achieve treatment goals and facilitate communication.

Stigma prevents many who need help from getting mental health care. Therapy dogs *Boe and Budge and the COSC dogs* pioneered a new role of the combat operational stress dog that improved morale and worked to destigmatize mental health intervention.

Today's therapy dogs and their human handlers integrate animal-assisted therapy into mainstream health care in a variety of settings and participate in studies to promote understanding of the benefits and outcomes of the human-animal bond. Today, Dog Pioneers of animal-assisted therapy help integrate contact with other living things into a highly technological health care system.

Seven Core Characteristics

Each dog pioneer of health care featured in this book was an individual. Each walked his own path. The dogs allowed the poetry of their gifts to emerge as they showed, helped, and taught their human partner by just doing what they were best at—being dogs.

These dogs changed health care directly and indirectly in various roles, in a variety of contexts, and in different ways. History called them to action, and each rose to meet the unique challenge of the time. They were different breeds, sizes, ages, and temperaments. However, they were more alike than they were different.

The dog pioneers of health care had seven defining characteristics.

1. *They were unexpected.* They surprised us. They were unknown, ordinary dogs who were on a "hero's journey. Many of the dogs and their human mentors shared a heroic narrative that had many attributes of the hero's journey described by Joseph Campbell.[2]

   They lived an ordinary life, waiting to be discovered, until they ventured from their ordinary worlds, and went into uncharted territory. Their human mentors introduced animals into a new role, or they stimulated a new vision of health care or both. The Pioneer dogs guided their human partners cross a new threshold into health care to inspire an innovative way of thinking about a health care process, need, or population. With their human mentors, the dogs encountered challenges, hardships, skepticism, tests, challenges, criticism, and doubt. But they rallied humans to action, changing humans' perspectives of what was possible. They became role models, heroic symbols, and metaphors as inspired humans shared the dogs' stories. Health care was changed by the new knowledge and experience brought to the world through human-animal collaboration.

2. *They found a human mentor.* The dog pioneers needed human partners. They found them in their human teachers and mentors. But these mentors not only taught and guided the dogs; they also

watched and learned from them. Edwin Richardson, Sigmund Freud, Boris Levinson, Florence Nightingale, Morris Frank, Leonhard Seppala, and the combat operational stress dog handlers paid attention to the dogs. They observed what dogs could do.

In turn, the dogs changed their mentor's view of what was possible. The dog pioneers showed them new ways to approach health and health care delivery. The relationships between the dogs and their human mentors were a triumph of the human-animal bond and partnership. The mentors understood their canine partners and allowed an interspecies collaboration to flourish. Their relationships fostered curiosity and exploration of the nature of the bond between humans and dogs and expanded human inquiry into how dogs could work in therapeutic settings.

3. *They were the right dog at a defining moment.* Each dog pioneer was called to action at his or her unique moment in history. They were the right dogs at the right time. The dogs' contributions rose out of human need: wars, need for health care reforms and social change, need for reformed ways of viewing and responding to public health needs, need for increased independence for disabled people, and need to reach out to those with mental illness.

4. *They had charm and charisma.* They got humans' attention. They showed up, and they were hard to ignore. From Jofi to Jingles to Buddy and Togo, their unique canine charm and appeal opened doors and made them an irresistible force. Each brought their unique gifts to the world and courageously met the challenge placed before them. Collies, bulldogs, shepherds, poodles, and retrievers all inspired us on the battlefield. A German shepherd at the other end of the leash with Morris Frank became a national symbol for independence for those who had disabilities. Balto and Togo, two very different dogsled dogs, created a new awareness of immunization when they conquered the most unforgiving of terrain.

Dog pioneers continue to amaze and inspire humans. Perhaps somewhere today a charming and gentle golden retriever sits at the side of a young cancer patient in the modern hospital and brings the poetry of the human-animal bond to the modern bedside.

5. *They raised our curiosity.* The dog pioneers made us wonder about the potential of the human-animal bond. Gradually, humans began to consider the role the human-animal collaboration might play in health care. What were the possibilities?

6. *They demonstrated what they could do.* Once they had our attention, they showed us what they could do, sometimes before humans asked

them or knew what they needed them to do. These trailblazing dogs worked their way into the consulting room, the battlefield, the Alaskan frontier, the streets of busy American cities, and the health care setting to teach unexpected lessons. In addition to the logical, scientific aspect of work with dogs, those who observed them carefully noticed and appreciated the *art* of what dogs could do at the intersection of human health. The dog pioneers showed humans the poetry of the healing comfort of the human-animal bond. They demonstrated the art of the dog as they worked gently with a troubled or injured child or silently comforted a troubled or dying soldier or steadfastly provided security and safety to a blind person as he crossed a dangerous city street.

7. *They made things better.* They innovated. How can a dog be an innovator? If these dogs changed health care, how did that happen? Improvements and innovations often come from unexpected places and in unexpected ways. How do changes move us in a different direction—especially in an environment as complex as health care?

Improvement requires change, and change involves creativity. Improvement, like the work of therapy dogs, is both an art and a science, both logical and artistic. To improve things, we need the logical part of our brains to form logical conclusions and the creative side of our brains to see the big picture—visualize new ideas and see the poetry of the human-animal bond.[3] To understand changes that are possible and implement them, both the science and the art of the therapy animal are needed, and perhaps this is what animals bring to improvement work. The Dog Pioneers helped us imagine new ways to help.

One way to innovate is by testing an idea on a small scale.[4] All process improvements require change, but not all changes are improvements, so someone has to test them. When someone tries a change and tests it, the change can be revised or modified if needed, and then the cycle can continue for ongoing improvement. This cycle of improvement characterized the work of the dog pioneers as the early innovators in animal-assisted interventions.

The dog pioneers were the innovators and early adopters of human-animal collaboration in health care. *Innovators* are those who want to be the first to try something. *Early adopters* come after innovators and represent opinion leaders who embrace change opportunities.

These dogs implemented change in small ways, with their mentors, testing it on a small scale, and then other early adopters of the change spread it or diffused it. These cycles of innovation and change still occur in animal-assisted intervention in health care. Today, study and testing and search for data and empirical evidence to support and understand the benefits of animal-assisted interventions continue, and health care providers are still learning how to best integrate these interventions into mainstream therapeutic care.

This type of change occurs in systems through a process known as diffusion of innovation. Understanding how diffusion of innovation works can help us understand why some in health care may be more likely than others to adopt AAI in health care as an innovation. Some may be early adopters of AAI, while others may wait for more evidence and diffusion of AAI as a health care modality.

Diffusion of innovation theory, developed by E. M. Rogers in 1962,[5] is a social science theory that explains how, over time, a new idea, improvement, or product gains momentum and diffuses (or spreads) through a system. The end result of this diffusion of change is that people, as part of a social system, adopt a new idea and do something differently. The key to adoption is that the person must perceive the idea, behavior, or product as new or innovative. This makes diffusion possible. However, adoption of a new idea or change does not happen simultaneously in a system. Some are more likely to adopt innovation than others.

Legacy: Mutuality and Connection

The dog pioneers blazed a path for a new generation of dogs in service to humans in health care. Thousands of new modern-day therapy dogs would follow them, walking through new doors into 21st-century mainstream health care. As more science became available to convince health care professionals of their merits, therapy dogs, their handlers, and providers began to learn more about how to integrate animal-assisted interventions into treatment plans, just as Boris Levinson had envisioned. New doors opened for a modern generation of dogs to show us what they could do in a human-animal partnership.

MUTUALITY

The legacy of the dog pioneers' contributions to health care is that they created human curiosity that spurred our ongoing quest to explore ways to increase our understanding of the mutuality of the human-animal bond and interspecies collaboration. The human-animal bond is a mutually beneficial and dynamic relationship between people and animals that is influenced by behaviors that are essential to the health and well-being of both.[6] Animals and humans occupy the same shared world and therefore have a common destiny. As humans have the privilege of working with our canine companions, it is logical that we have a responsibility and opportunity to appreciate the mutuality of the human-animal bond. When humans ask dogs to perform human work and dogs do so out of their canine devotion, a fundamental part of that collaboration is discerning and responding to what humans may owe dogs in return.

What does this reciprocity look like when it comes to our working relationship with dogs? It entails consideration for the safety and welfare of the dogs who serve us out of their devotion, including evaluation of the suitability and type of experience the dog will have. When animals are engaged for any human purpose, an ethical obligation exists to ensure their health and well-being.[7] We must serve as an advocate for our working animals, be able to recognize their stress and understand their communication, behavior, emotions, interactions, and personalities, and know how to keep them safe from injury.[8]

While animal-assisted interventions are designed to be beneficial to humans, they must be balanced with provisions for the safety and welfare of the therapy animal.[9] The effect of animal-assisted interventions for humans is becoming more evident in scientific studies, but the impact of these interventions on the well-being of the animals has not been well understood or researched. Although many handlers in animal-assisted interventions enthusiastically claim the animals enjoy the work, it's not clear from the documented evidence that this is so. The benefits to the animals are not self-evident. In 2017, McCullough and colleagues studied the physiological and behavioral effects of animal-assisted interventions on 26 therapy dog handler teams at five children's hospitals in pediatric oncology settings and found that dogs did not have increased stress-associated behaviors during intervention sessions.[10] The effect of the animal-assisted intervention on therapy dogs needs further empirical study to validate these findings. The ability to view dogs as sentient beings with feelings is a prerequisite to being able to learn the lessons they can teach us.

Our reciprocal relationship with our canine partners requires that we respect who they are. They are not little humans or objects, but a unique species with talents, needs, and behaviors that are both helpful and mysterious to us. They are not capable of volunteering for dangerous tasks but freely do so out of a willingness to please us. To fully appreciate our collaborative work with dogs, it seems fitting that we should appreciate, understand, and celebrate their canine nature and expect only that of them. An essential part of understanding other animals is taking time to listen to their messages to us and to learn from the stories of those who spend their lives living and working with another species. Studies have shown that when humans can empathize with animals, they can translate that into human-directed empathy.[11]

One of our responsibilities for living in the world with our dogs is to understand the ethical and moral conflicts that arise when we put them in harm's way to perform our work. We can't assume our dogs "love the work" if we have not begun to understand their language, signals, and ways of telling us they are stressed, tired, or not suitable for the work we have assigned them. Our dogs often show us the roles they want and can do. Like Togo who showed his leadership and Bellin who demonstrated his ability to comfort even the most vulnerable, our dogs lead the way if we listen and pay attention. Understanding our dog's behavior involves being educated on dog behavior, signs of stress, and the basis of animal behavior such as signals dogs use to calm themselves when stressed. Understanding these "calming signals" may help dog handlers better understand their dog's communication and know when to remove the dog from a stressful situation.[12] A handler can then take action if the dog appears to be stressed. Humans have an obligation to provide for the wellness and safety of animals involved in animal-assisted interventions.[13]

The concept of animal welfare was expressed in the Five Freedoms for animals that were developed in the Bramble Report.[14] They were designed in response to a 1965 United Kingdom government report on livestock husbandry and were formalized in 1979 by the UK Farm Animal Welfare Council. The Five Freedoms are internationally accepted standards of practice that assert a living being's right to humane treatment.[15] The Five Freedoms outline five aspects of animal welfare under human control:

1. Freedom from hunger and thirst
2. Freedom from discomfort
3. Freedom from pain, injury, or disease
4. Freedom to express normal behavior
5. Freedom from fear and distress

Animal welfare means "how an animal is coping with the conditions in which it lives."[16] According to this concept, an animal's primary welfare needs can be met by providing the five freedoms. Violations of these freedoms cause animals to stress and negatively impact their welfare. The Five Freedoms have been adopted by professional groups including veterinarians and organizations including the World Organization for Animal Health.[17]

However, therapy animals have needs beyond the Five Freedoms.[18] Mellor noted that the Five Freedoms have limitations because they focus on animals' freedom from a negative perspective and that animal welfare should focus on positive experiences for the animals.[19] Five provisions were proposed, aligned with the Five Freedoms, that promoted positive welfare management. Tedeschi suggested the capability approach, which provides a theoretical framework for animal entitlements, and suggested compassionate relationships, including the right to flourish.[20] According to the model, animals should have a wide range of capabilities to function, including bodily health and integrity, an opportunity to play, and control of their environment, and these guidelines go beyond the Five Freedoms.[21]

Other organizations have also provided guidelines for the welfare of animals involved in animal-assisted interventions. The International Association of Human-Animal Interaction Organizations' definitions for animal-assisted intervention and guidelines for the wellness of animals outline ethical practice for the well-being of the animals involved.[22] Humans have a job to do in our relationship with canine partners. The work of a human in the human-animal partnership is to care for and provide food, shelter, health care, safety, physical activity, and mental stimulation for the animal.

CONNECTION AND ONE HEALTH

The Dog Pioneers also raised humans' awareness of our connectedness to animals. As humans interacted with the Dog Pioneers, we became aware of the different ways dogs, and humans can contribute to the well-being of each other. Today, in an increasingly technological world, dogs and other animals bring us the opportunity to connect—with our own species and with others. This connection is essential to our health, well-being, and comfort.

Our connections with animals are deep and significant. The fate of animals and humans depends on each other. We occupy the same planet. In a world where we are all so connected, we have a mutual need and responsibility to care for each other and respect the unique gifts of each species. This extends from biology to psychology to public health and society to symbols and healing. We are just discovering what we can learn from our animal companions, about them and about ourselves.

Interest in human-animal interaction and the mental life of animals has increased in those who have the opportunity to observe other species. The emotional life of animals, once dismissed as anthropomorphic, is gaining greater acceptance. Works such as Temple Grandin's books *Animals Make Us Human* and *Animals in Translation,* as well as others,[23] have proposed a connection between human intelligence and animal intelligence and suggested that animals demonstrate behavior and thinking that resemble regret, shame, guilt, revenge, and love. Grandin said she didn't know all the talents animals possess—or how they could apply their talents if we gave them a chance. She added, "I'm willing to bet that just about any dog can remember where you put your car keys better than you can if you're over forty, and probably if you're under forty too."[24]

In our world, the health of animals, humans, and the environment is interconnected.[25] Barbara Natterson-Horowitz, M.D., is a coauthor of the book *Zoobiquity* that describes the connection between human and animal health.

Natterson-Horowitz wrote that she developed the concepts of interspecies connectedness to improve her work as a physician and looked to animals for answers to human health issues because of our species' shared vulnerabilities.[26]

The interconnectedness of animals and human health is being increasingly integrated into one approach to a healthy world. *One Health* is "a worldwide strategy for expanding interdisciplinary collaborations and communications in all aspects of health care for humans, animals, and the environment."[27] The concept that the health of people is connected to that of animals and the environment is the foundation of the One Health Initiative, a collaborative approach that works at the local, national, and global level.[28] The goal of the One Health Initiative is to achieve optimal health outcomes by recognizing the interconnectedness between people, animals, and their shared environment. This effort requires the collaboration of multiple disciples—human health care, veterinary professionals, and environmentalists—promoting strengths in leadership and management.[29]

The term "One Health" or "One Medicine" is not new but has become more important as changes have occurred in interactions between humans, animals, and the environment. Dr. Calvin Schwabe, a founding faculty member of the University of California at Davis School of Medicine as well as an epidemiology professor at the School of Veterinary Medicine, coined the term "One Medicine" in his 1964 book, *Veterinary Medicine and Human Health*.[30] The Centers for Disease Control and Prevention established its One Health Office in 2009, advancing the concept globally, recognizing that public health interventions require the cooperation of human-animal and environmental communities.[31]

From medic, triage, and transport, from muse to metaphor, and from therapy to service as the dog pioneers worked by the side of their human mentors, they were examples of interspecies collaboration that affected human health. Their contributions showed that animals and humans could collaborate in innovative ways to improve health care.

New Pioneers and Possibilities

So now, we ask, what can a new generation of pioneering dogs show us? A new generation will step forth over the next decades to reveal innovative ways that the human animal partnership can help humans find ways to create healthy communities for both animals and people. As technology increasingly becomes a delivery vehicle for health care, the potential grows for the art and science of human-animal bond to contribute to our understanding of how to deliver high touch and highly technical health care. The opportunities for cross-species collaboration and learning are likely to be vast and varied.

CROSS-SPECIES COLLABORATION, INNOVATION AND RESEARCH

Research into canine disease and illnesses may open new ways to understand human health and diseases such as cancer. We will discover more ways in which dog and human health are related. Dogs and other animals may teach us about human health, disease and how to prevent and treat it. Roles for dogs are evolving in detecting human illnesses such as cancer in tissue samples, fluctuations in blood sugar or seizures. Researchers from human and veterinary medicine learn more by studying across species and now can combine scientific findings to benefit both humans and animals by studying cancers shared by humans and dogs.

In mental health services, as we study the learning capabilities and skills of our canine partners, they may show us new approaches to counseling, reducing the stigma of asking for mental health services.

THERAPY DOGS AND ASSISTANCE DOGS

There will continue to be a demand for therapy dogs and a demand for increased standards to guide their work. Health care organizations and professionals of the future, provided with more valid and reliable studies about the impact of animal-assisted interventions in health care, will consider the human-animal bond as part of their toolkit of health care interventions. Dogs that can detect seizures or cancer may show us how they can add to health care prevention and treatment. Dogs in assistance and service roles will continue to show us new ways the human-canine partnership can provide increased independence for those with disabilities. Dogs are already assisting those who have disabilities such as sight or hearing impairments, but the next generation of pioneer dogs may show us new ways that people can learn how to live more independently when assisted by a dog.

BUILDING HEALTHY COMMUNITIES

Future dog pioneers may help us build health communities by understanding how to prevent violence to living things. If humans listen and pay attention, perhaps the next generation of pioneer dogs will be messengers who speak volumes to us about prevention of violence against living things and the link between animal abuse and human violence.

Building healthy communities means creating a place where everyone is safe. When animals are abused, humans are often at risk. Lessons from dogs and other companion animals, who are often our most vulnerable family members, can inform what we know about violence prevention. Animal cruelty does not occur in isolation; it may be the "the tip of the iceberg "of a pattern of human violence. Animal abuse does not occur in isolation. It is one form of interrelated family violence and dysfunction. Increasing evidence has shown strong links between animal cruelty and other crimes, including interpersonal, family and community violence.[32]

Abuse of an animal can be an early predictor of future or concurrent violent acts and a "red flag" warning signal ad the first opportunity for social service or law enforcement to intervene. The earlier the cycle of violence is interrupted, the higher the chance of successful intervention. No longer is the family pet viewed with the old attitude of "It's just an animal. Instead, awareness is growing of humans and dogs and other companion pets as an interspecies family whose safety and destiny are linked.[33]

Complex societal problems such as violence require complex solutions. Through an increased understanding of risks to companion animals through the interspecies cycles of violence and recognition of animal abuse as a significant dynamic, professionals can move to the protection of all vulnerable member of society. "The Link" is a term used to describe the intersection between animal cruelty, child maltreatment, domestic violence, and elder abuse. The National Link Coalition is an informal, multidisciplinary, collaborative network of individuals and organizations in human services and animal welfare who address the intersections between animal abuse, domestic violence, child maltreatment, and elder abuse through research, public policy, programming, and community awareness. The groups believe that human and animal well-being are inextricably intertwined and that the prevention of family and community violence can best be achieved through partnerships representing multi-species perspectives.[34]

The Dog Pioneers of tomorrow will appear with creativity and innovation and will show us exciting things about themselves and ourselves. While we wait for more empirical studies to further prove the benefit of the human-animal bond in health care, our dogs will be busy showing us the way. Hopefully, we will watch and listen to the art, science, and poetry of our dogs as they show and tell us their stories. With the legacy of the Dog Pioneers of health care inspiring us, we can walk into the future of health care with dogs by our sides as we search for ways to

- Improve animal and human health locally, nationally, and globally
- Understand and encourage interspecies learning in health care
- Develop sound foundations in the reciprocity of the human-animal bond by better understanding the impact our work together has on our dogs and our dogs' communication

- Add to scientific knowledge about the benefits of the human-animal bond and animal-assisted interventions in health care through quantitative and qualitative, uniform and rigorous scientific study
- Increase use of a standards-based approach and common terminology in animal-assisted therapy
- Develop valid and reliable process and outcome measurement tools and outcome logic models for animal-assisted intervention programs in health care
- Integrate education on the human-animal bond into health professionals' training
- Share our dogs' stories and factually communicate both the art and science of their work

Over the decades, the Dog Pioneers stepped in to show us how they could contribute to health care in ways we had not envisioned. Throughout history, a few special humans were there who watched and understood. The Dog Pioneers left us a legacy of partnership with dogs and an ongoing quest for learning about the possibilities of the human-animal bond. We need to understand, study, and imagine what more interspecies collaboration can do. New doors of opportunity for increased mutuality and interspecies collaboration in health care are opening, and we are walking through them with our dogs. As we consider how the Dog Pioneers led us to unexpected discoveries, it is tantalizing to think where the next Dog Pioneers in health care may lead us.

Not every dog is a pioneer. But the common characteristics of the Dog Pioneers show us that the face of the Dog Pioneer is the face of the hero. Their work as medics, muse, myths and health care pioneers shows us that some dogs can indeed change the world.

Epilogue

The relationship between a dog and a human is always complicated. The two know each other in a way nobody else quite understands, a connection shrouded in personal history, temperament, experience, instinct, and love.— Jon Katz[1]

If you have ever loved a dog, you will not be surprised that I can't let you get away without at least one more story about my own dog, Junior. It is only fitting because it was Junior who started me on the journey to write this book and who sat below my desk with his head on my knee as I told the stories of the Dog Pioneers. Junior has been my pioneer dog—showing me how to blaze my new path in the second act of my life.

This book has been about what dogs show us about their ability to help people and ourselves and how they do so. It has also been a tribute to my own journey of self-discovery as I learned about myself from Junior and the other dogs with whom I have had the privilege to share my life's journey. So here's what I've learned : when you tell a dog story, you really tell your own story. Dogs show us ourselves in compelling ways. We look at our dogs and see the best in ourselves.

When I first heard the story of the Mercy Dogs, Freud and Jofi, Levinson and Jingles, I was not at all surprised that these clever dogs changed their human partners. I wasn't surprised because it had happened to me.

It was July, the middle of a sweltering Texas summer. My husband, George, and I were grieving. Max, our golden retriever, had just died of cancer. Max had been with us for 15 years and died just as the three of us began our new world of retirement.

Now that Max was gone, it was my husband and me, trying to figure out what was next. The house was filled with lonely silence, but the empty dog bowls still in their place spoke volumes. No dog toys littered the rooms; no

160

one woke me with a wet nose asking to be let out at 6:00 a.m. We slept later now but would have gladly risen at 6:00 to answer a golden retriever's wake-up call.

People handle grief in many ways. George, my husband of almost 50 years, vowed never to have a dog again.

"Never again. It hurts too much. No more dogs," he said.

But I knew I needed another dog. And soon. I was a volunteer with our local golden retriever rescue, and it was hard to see homeless goldens come and go almost daily.

"Let's foster a golden," I told George.

"No way."

I tried again: "Just to have a dog in the house again."

"No, you know that dog will never leave."

Two days later, on a 100-degree Texas Saturday, I saw a rescued young red golden retriever arrive when I volunteered at the rescue adoption day. He had been pulled from a busy shelter just before his time ran out to be adopted.

I watched that skinny red dog jump up, sloppily kiss a prospective adopter, and almost knock her down. He barked every time someone tried to speak. He lunged so hard on the leash he nearly knocked me over when I tried to untangle the flustered adopter from the leash that had wrapped around both her feet and the feet of the somersaulting dog. The woman caught her breath, adjusted her crisp white blouse, smoothed out her wrinkled white linen shorts, and looked down with disdain at the red dynamo.

"No, he's too red and too wild. Are you sure he's even a real golden retriever? He is so red he looks like an Irish setter." The red golden retriever and I stared at each other, but neither of us answered her question. We just panted.

I saw little beads of perspiration begin to form and drip the prospective adopter's flawless cake makeup down her face. Her perfectly coiffed, blonde highlighted Texas "big hair" was wilting fast in the Texas heat and now looked to me as flat as a big brown cow patty against her head. The dripping woman quickly turned her attention to a large, docile, mature, light blonde female golden. That big girl golden sat munching a carrot snack under the shade of a live oak tree. She was freshly groomed golden retriever in all her glory, gorgeous, and serene. The dog looked like she might have been meditating.

In less than an hour, I saw two blonde heads, one human and one canine, sitting with perfect posture, driving off together in the front seat of their air-conditioned Lexus. Meanwhile, the rejected red wild golden still next to me was not discouraged. He put both paws on my shoulder, licked the pouring sweat off my face, looked me in the eyes, and flashed a golden retriever grin.

"Okay, I will foster him until he finds a home." I was astonished to hear those words coming out of my mouth.

The foster coordinator looked at both of us, grinned, and handed me the leash. I hung on to that leash with all my strength as my new foster dog pulled me to my waiting car. I lurched in and pushed my new charge's bouncing red, golden retriever rear end towards my car and loaded him into my yellow VW Beetle. Sweat poured down my back and face. We both landed in the back seat and again grinned at each other. I worked on a plan to get us both into the front seat and to introduce our new houseguest to George when we got home.

After a week, George and I adopted the red golden. I worried about raising this new boy because he was so unlike our docile, sweet Max. But I suspected this young, energetic, and bright golden now named Junior was just what two newly retired boomers needed. We were in search of new purpose and projects in retirement and, without Max, we felt lost. It didn't take long for Junior to show us the way, and all three of us began the work on our second acts.

Junior became a registered therapy dog, and I became a registered therapy dog handler. When I began working with Junior as a therapy dog, I knew the experience would be rewarding for me, and I hoped for him. As Junior and I visited children in libraries and read books with them and visited children in play therapy sessions, I was amazed at the communication connections that occurred. As a health care professional, I was surprised and moved at how transformational the relationship between dog and human could be. I saw firsthand the art and science and the poetry of animal-assisted intervention.

When we joined a play therapist and child in a therapy session, I sat in silence on the blanket or in a chair close to Junior. The therapist was always present in the room and guided the therapy session. Children who had previously been noncommunicative would talk to Junior. Some brushed his hair. I was reminded of how Jingles and Levinson had worked together. Gradually the therapist entered into the conversation between Junior and the child as the talking and playing continued. The child would tell the therapist what he or she thought Junior might be thinking. One child braided the hair on Junior's long golden tail while Junior closed his eyes and the child described what she thought Junior might be dreaming about.

One weekday afternoon, we were in a community center reading with young, struggling readers after school, a type of informal animal-assisted activity. The sound of the child reading is the cue for Junior to quietly go to a "down" position. He works on his red fleece blanket embroidered with a big pawprint and the name JUNIOR in all caps. Junior's job, in addition to listening to the reader, no matter how many words are imperfectly pronounced, is to save the place in the book by placing his paw on the page when given the "paw-stay" command. Junior holds the place in the book if the child reading to him wants to ask Junior questions about the story. Often the child answers for the dog. We find out what both Junior and the child think about the story. Junior often gets so relaxed, he rolls over to invite a belly rub. Sometimes the big golden retriever even dozes off. When the occasional nap happens, I explain that Junior is closing his eyes to dream about the story; usually, all but the most skeptical readers go along with the fantasy of the dreaming golden retriever.

One day, the session was held in a cozy nook at an after-school program in a community center. We were surrounded by bright green and yellow books as the sun streamed into the room. A boy with a crisp white shirt and school uniform slacks appeared for his turn to read with the dog, nodded a quick hello, carried a book, and sat right on the blanket's pawprint. The boy had not been smiling until now. The sunlight streaming through the window got brighter and shined in my eyes. I saw that the child had a few crumbs left on his shirt from his after-school snack. I gave Junior a gentle command, "leave it," as I saw Junior spot the cookie crumbs.

The boy wiggled back on the blanket, just out of Junior's reach, giggled softly, and then moved forward, smiling, to rest gently on the reclining big red dog. The boy placed one tentative hand on Junior's paw and began to struggle to read slowly, almost in a whisper, turning the book around to face the dog and to point out the picture of a red dog. Junior nosed the page in interest, and all three of us entered the story.[2]

I had been struggling with a newly diagnosed chronic illness that altered my ability to physically do many things I enjoyed. Along with that came feelings of loss, sadness, and discouragement. I often wanted to stop trying. When I saw Junior connect with others who were also struggling, I saw, through him, what drawing comfort and joy and courage from each moment meant.

As I watched my dog interact with struggling readers, it reminded me of how much better I felt when I interacted with Junior. I was curious. In spite of how sad or discouraged I was struggling with chronic illness, why did I feel better when I spent time with my dog? What was it about his connection to others that touched them? Why did it inspire and comfort me? What was happening during the human-animal interaction? What was Junior feeling during these encounters?

Watching a therapy dog at work can make abstract concepts like resilience, generosity, and service come to life. Because therapy animals cannot use words, they demonstrate rather than tell us about their qualities. When I worked with Junior, a rescued dog who spent his first year living most days in a crate, I saw how rescued dogs don't look back on their troubled past but enjoy their work every day. And I saw that the time the therapy dog spends on each visit is a special gift to each person, including the human at the other end of the leash.

Junior taught me about gratitude and starting over. He showed me there is always a "Plan B." I saw that, although I could no longer do many physical activities I used to do, I could still work with my therapy dog. Junior showed me how to make the best of life. We both still had gifts to give; I could still contribute. I realized that giving my time to someone is an excellent gift. For me, the path to my own resilience was through service to others. My dog showed me the way. I was grateful.

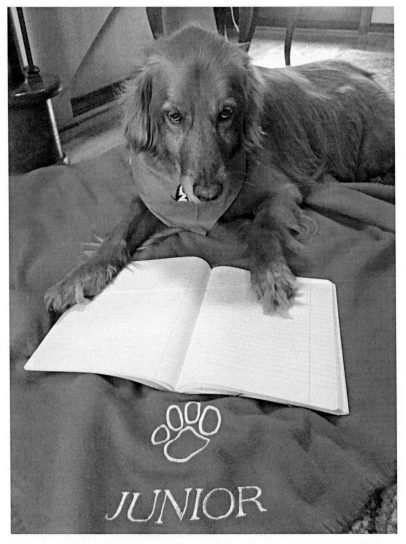

Junior, a registered therapy dog, holds a place with a "Paw-stay" as he waits for a young reader, 2014 (photograph by Jill Schilp, courtesy *The Daily Junior Blog*).

Junior taught me courage and resilience. I learned not to give up on my goals, even if I am not successful the first time. When we volunteered as a therapy dog team, Junior and I shared his story of how he had to study to pass his therapy dog test and didn't give up when he wasn't ready to pass the first time. It was another lesson: ask for and get help if you need it.

I watched Junior visit children and adults who struck up conversations with the friendly dog, and I learned that it feels good when someone listens to you and asks you what you need, and it helps to tell someone what you need.

Dogs like Junior are becoming integrated into health care treatment plans, just as Boris Levinson had envisioned. Perhaps new Dog Pioneers will follow them to show us more about the integration of the two parts of living creatures' nature, the logical and the poetic.

Our dogs walk into the hearts of their human guardians, never to leave that sacred space where the human-animal bond resides. I still believe that dogs can change the world. If we watch them, they will show us the way, and we will continue to tell their stories.

What's your dog's story?

Glossary

Affect   Any experience of feeling or emotion.[1]

Animal-assisted activity (AAA)   A planned and goal-oriented informal interaction and visitation conducted by the human-animal team for motivational, educational, and recreational purposes.[2]

Animal-assisted education (AAE)   A goal-directed planned and structured intervention delivered by educational and related service professionals.[3]

Animal-assisted intervention (AAI)   A goal-oriented and structured intervention that intentionally includes or incorporates animals in health, education, or human service (e.g., social work) for the purpose of therapeutic gains in humans.[4]

Animal-assisted therapy (AAT)   A goal-directed, planned, and structured therapeutic intervention directed and/or delivered by health, education and human service professionals. AAT is delivered and included in the professional documentation. AAT is delivered and/or directed by a formally trained (with active licensure, degree or equivalent) professional with expertise within the scope of the professionals' practice.[5]

Assistance dogs   A broad term used to describe dogs that have been individually trained to do work or perform tasks for an individual with a disability. Assistance animals are also commonly called "service" animals. The tasks performed by the dog must be directly related to the person's disability. Examples include guide dogs for people who are blind, hearing dogs for people who are deaf, and dogs who provide mobility assistance or communicate medical alerts. Assistance dogs are considered working animals, not pets.[6]

Blindness   Legal blindness is the sight of 20/200 or worse in the better eye with the best possible correction, or a visual field (peripheral vision) of 20 degrees or less. It is possible to be legally blind and still be able to read, see colors, perceive light, or recognize faces.[7]

Child psychotherapy   A variety of techniques and methods used to help children and adolescents who are experiencing difficulties with their emotions or behavior.[8]

Co-therapist   One of two therapists working with a client, a pair of clients, or a couple, family, or group to enhance understanding and to change behavior and relationships during treatment.[9]

Countertransference   The analyst's or therapist's unconscious and conscious feelings and attitudes towards the patient and his or her reaction to the patient's transference.[10]

Diffusion of innovation   A social science theory developed by E. M. Rogers in 1962 that explains how, over time, a new idea, improvement, or product gains momentum and diffuses (or spreads) through a system. The result of this diffusion of change is that people, as part of a social system, adopt a new idea and do something differently.[11]

Diphtheria   An infection caused by the bacterium *Corynebacterium diphtheriae.* Diphtheria causes a thick covering in the back of the throat. It can lead to difficulty breathing, heart failure, paralysis, and even death.[12]

Diphtheria antitoxin   A treatment for diphtheria in the United States first used the 1890s.[13]

Emotional support dog   A pet that provides therapeutic support to a person with mental illness. An emotional support dog must be prescribed by a licensed mental health professional. Emotional support animals do not have the same rights to public access as service dogs.[14]

Facility dog   A dog who is regularly present in a residential or clinical setting. The facility dog might live with a handler who is an employee of the facility and come to work each day, or might live at the facility full time under the care of a primary staff person. Facility dogs should be specially trained for extended interactions with clients or residents of the facility.[15]

Foment   To treat with moist heat as for easing pain.[16]

Free association   The process whereby the patient tells the story of his or her life by just saying whatever comes to mind.[17]

Guide dog   An assistance dog who has been trained to assist a blind or visually impaired person.

Human-animal bond   A mutually beneficial and dynamic relationship between people and animals that is influenced by behaviors essential to the health and well-being of both.[18]

Humane   Having or showing a compassionate benevolence for people, animals, and the environment and recognizing the interdependence of all living things.

Immunization   A process by which a person becomes protected against disease through vaccination. This term is often used interchangeably with vaccination or inoculation and is also used to mean the act of introducing a vaccine into the body to produce immunity to a specific disease.[19]

Infection control   Infection control is the policies, procedures, and practices that prevent or stop the spread of infections in health care settings.

The Link   A term used to describe the intersection between animal cruelty, child maltreatment, domestic violence and elder abuse.[30]

Meta-analysis   A quantitative, formal, statistical analysis used to systematically assess previous research studies to derive conclusions about that body of research. Outcomes from a meta-analysis may include a more precise estimate of the effect of treatment or risk factor for disease, or other outcomes, than any individual study contributing to the pooled analysis.[20]

Metaphor   A figure of speech in which a word or a phrase literally denoting one kind of object or idea is used in place of another to suggest an object, activity or idea.[21]

Occupational therapy   The use of everyday activities with individuals and groups for the purpose of participation in roles and situations at home, school, the workplace, community, and other settings. Occupational therapy is provided for rehabilitation and promotion of health and wellness to those who have or are at risk for developing an illness, disease, condition, disorder, impairment, or limitation.[22]

One Health   The integrative effort of multiple disciplines working together to obtain optimum health for people, animals, and the environment. It recognizes that the health of each is connected to the others.[23]

Outcome   Results or effects of a program.

Outcome logic model   A graphical description of the relationship between the inputs, outputs, goals, processes, objectives, and outcomes of a program. Outcome models provide a picture of how a program is intended to work and are helpful in program evaluation.

Oxytocin   A hormone produced in the brain that promotes feelings of attachment. It plays an essential role in social bonding and bonding between mothers and infants and has a role in socialization and stress relief. It is often called the "love hormone."

Pet therapy   A term widely used several decades ago to refer to animal training programs and animal-assisted interventions. The preferred terms adopted today by many therapy organizations are animal-assisted intervention, animal-assisted activity, and animal-assisted therapy.[24]

Pioneer   One who goes before to prepare the way for others to follow.

Process   Activities and outputs of a program.

Psychoanalysis   An approach to the mind, personality, psychological disorders, and psychological treatment originally developed by Sigmund Freud at the beginning of the 20th century. The hallmark of psychoanalysis is the assumption that much mental activity is unconscious, and that understanding people requires interpreting the unconscious meaning underlying their overt behavior.[25]

Psychotherapy   Any psychological service provided by a trained professional that primarily uses forms of communication and interaction to assess, diagnose, and treat dysfunctional emotional reactions, ways of thinking, and behavior patterns.[26]

Repression   A defense where an individual's impulses and instinctual desires are blocked from consciousness. It is a process of unconsciously blocking ideas or memories that are viewed as unacceptable.[27]

Resistance   A patient's unconscious opposition to exploring painful memories or content during psychoanalysis, during which the patient tells the story of his or her life by just saying whatever comes to mind.[28]

Service dog   See *Assistance dog.*

Stigma   A phenomenon that occurs when one person or group views another in a negative way because the person has a certain distinguishing trait. Negative attitudes and beliefs toward people who have a mental health problem are common.[29]

Therapy   Remediation of physical, medical, or behavioral disorders or disease.[31]

Therapy dogs   Dogs that visit with a handler to provide affection and comfort to various members of the public, typically in a variety of facility settings such as hospitals, retirement homes, and schools. Therapy dog teams pass a test by a national organization that shows the handler and the animal are suitable. Therapy dog teams are volunteers, and the dogs are personal pets. They are used as part of a treatment program in animal-assisted therapy, or in less formal, social activity as animal-assisted activity.[32]

Transference   In psychoanalysis, a patient's projection onto another person (the analyst) of feelings, past associations, experiences, and wishes originally associated with important individuals such as parents. In a broader context, an unconscious repetition of earlier behaviors and their projection onto new subjects. Transference has a recognized role in therapeutic encounters. It is important because it demonstrates that experiences affect the present, and interpreting transference in the psychoanalytic setting can shed light on unresolved conflicts.[33]

Triage   The screening and classification of casualties to maximize the survival and welfare of patients and to make the best use of treatment resources.[34]

Vaccine   A product that stimulates a person's immune system to produce immunity to a specific disease, protecting the person from that disease.[35]

Chapter Notes

Introduction

1. American Veterinary Medical Association, "Human-Animal Bond."
2. Schilp, "Is Your Dog's Gaze the Look of Love?"
3. Nagasawa et al., "Oxytocin-Gaze Positive Loop"; MacClean and Hare, "Dogs Hijack the Human Bonding Pathway."
4. Nagasawa et al., "Oxytocin-Gaze Positive Loop."
5. Pet Partners, "Terminology."
6. *Ibid.*
7. *Ibid.*

Chapter 1

1. Jager, *Scout, Red Cross and Army Dogs*, 2–7.
2. *Ibid.*
3. *Ibid.*
4. Correa, "The Dog's Sense of Smell."
5. Jager, *Scout, Red Cross and Army Dogs*, 6.
6. U.S. War Dogs Association, "World War I."
7. Richardson, *British War Dogs: Their Training and Psychology*, 124.
8. *Ibid.*, 50.
9. *Ibid.*, 52.
10. *Ibid.*, 57.
11. *Ibid.*, 53.
12. *Ibid.*, 64–82.
13. Frankel, "The Dog Whisperer."
14. *Ibid.*
15. Jager, *Scout, Red Cross and Army Dogs*, 15–21.
16. "Triage," Tabers Medical Dictionary (https://www.tabers.com/tabersonline/view/Tabers-Dictionary/735812/all/triage).

17. Pollock, 'Triage and Management of the Injured in World War I."
18. Cox, "Dogs of War: The First Aiders on Four Legs."
19. Jones, "Shell Shocked."
20. *Ibid.*
21. Pols and Oak, "War and Military Mental Health." For more information on shell shock, see Leese, *Shell Shock*.
22. Richardson, *British War Dogs*, 60.
23. "Red Cross Dogs," The Literary Digest.
24. Baynes, "Our Animal Allies in the World War."
25. Hendrick, "Merciful Dogs of War."
26. Prasad, *Caesar, the Anzac Dog.*
27. "Stubby of A.E.F. Enters Valhalla," *New York Times.*
28. Bausum, *Sergeant Stubby.*
29. Richardson, *British War Dogs: Their Training and Psychology*, 60.
30. *Ibid.*, 66.
31. Dyer, "Wanted: More Red Cross Dogs for America."
32. "No More Dogs Needed Please," *Red Cross Magazine.*
33. American Veterinary Medical Association, "Human-Animal Bond."
34. Rosa, "Battling Canine Post-Traumatic Stress Disorder."
35. Richardson, *British War Dogs: Their Training and Psychology,* 177.

Chapter 2

1. The description of Freud's office is based on Hilda Doolittle's description which appears in Hilda Doolittle, *Tribute to Freud,* 1–17 and Friedman, *Analyzing Freud,* xiii–xv.
2. Friedman, *Analyzing Freud,* 31.
3. Doolittle, *Tribute to Freud,* 95.

4. *Ibid.*

5. Doolittle's *Tribute to Freud* and her letters and accounts provide the richest and most detailed description of the analysis process and Jofi's central role in it. Most of Freud's biographers and accounts of Freud's colleagues, friends, patients, and family include comments about Jofi and Freud's other dogs playing a central role in his life. See Genosko's Introduction to *Topsy*; Jones, *The Life and Work of Sigmund Freud*; Gay, *Freud: A Life for Our Time*; Edmundson, *The Death of Sigmund Freud*; Martin Freud, *Glory Reflected: Sigmund Freud—Man and Father*; Friedman, *Analyzing Freud*; and Grinker, "Reminiscences of a Personal Contact with Freud."

6. Doolittle, *Tribute to Freud*, 1.

7. *Ibid.*, 55.

8. Molnar, "Of Dogs and Doggerel."

9. Green, "Freud's Dream Companions."

10. For a more comprehensive review of Freud, his life and work and the development of Freudian therapy, see Jones, *The Life and Work of Sigmund Freud*; Gay, *Freud: A Life for Our Time*; Edmundson, *The Death of Sigmund Freud*; Martin Freud, *Glory Reflected: Sigmund Freud—Man and Father*; and Friedman, *Analyzing Freud*. For a more comprehensive discussion of psychoanalytical theory, practice, and history see Mitchell and Black, *Freud and Beyond*.

11. As quoted in Gay, *Freud: A Life for Our Time*, 592–593.

12. Friedman, *Analyzing Freud*, xiv.

13. Chandler, *Animal-Assisted Therapy in Counseling*, 150.

14. Edmundson, *The Death of Sigmund Freud*, 1117.

15. *Ibid.*

16. American Psychoanalytic Association, "Psychoanalytic Terms."

17. The couch, associated with the public image of psychoanalysis, is no longer required. Some psychoanalysts use the couch while some clinicians feel a face-to-face environment works best.

18. American Psychoanalytic Association, "Psychoanalytic Terms."

19. *Ibid.*

20. Quote attributed to Sigmund Freud in Anna Freud, "Foreword."

21. Edmundson, *The Death of Sigmund Freud*, 1073.

22. Freud quoted in Edmundson, *The Death of Sigmund Freud*, 1073, and Braitman, "Dog Complex: Analyzing Freud's Relationship with His Pets."

23. Anna's dog Wolf died in 1936, and in 1937 Jofi had ovarian costs removed and died of a heart attack 3 days later.

24. Edmundson, *The Death of Sigmund Freud*, 1043.

25. Chowtales, "Why Did Chows Change?"

26. H. D. Letter to Bryher, March 10, 1933, in Freidman, *Analyzing Freud*, 69.

27. Chow Chow Club, "A Chow's Personality and Habits"; Chowtales, "Why Did Chows Change?"

28. H. D. Letter to Conrad Aiken, August 26, 1933, in Friedman, *Analyzing Freud*, 371.

29. HD and Bryher papers.

30. *Ibid.*

31. Hilda Doolittle's letters, which appear in Friedman, *Analyzing Freud*, provide a rich account of Freud's clinical practice and provided the source of information about Hilda Doolittle's description of Jofi and the dog's role in her analysis (see xiii, 31, 50, 59, 69, 96, 141, 292, 331, and 371).

32. Phillips, "Introduction."

33. Holland, "H. D.'s Analysis with Freud."

34. Friedman, *Analyzing Freud*, 35, 59, 141, 371; Genosko, "Introduction"; Doolittle, *Tribute to Freud*, 95–97, 114, 145; Phillips, *Becoming Freud*.

35. Genosko, "Introduction."

36. Gay, *Freud: A Life for Our Time*, 12–14; Jones, *The Life and Work of Sigmund Freud*; Edmundson, *The Death of Sigmund Freud*; Martin Freud, *Glory Reflected: Sigmund Freud—Man and Father*; Friedman, *Analyzing Freud*; Grinker, "My Father's Analysis with Sigmund Freud"; Grinker, "Reminiscences of a Personal Contact with Freud"; Genosko, "Introduction."

37. Showalter, "Freud's Damn Dog."

38. Grinker, "My Father's Analysis with Sigmund Freud"; Grinker, "Reminiscences of a Personal Contact with Freud"; Gay, *Freud: A Life for Our Time*, 12–14; Showalter, "Freud's Damn Dog."

39. Grinker, "My Father's Analysis with Sigmund Freud"; Grinker, "Reminiscences of a Personal Contact with Freud."

40. Doolittle, *Tribute to Freud*, 160.

41. *Ibid.*

42. Braitman, "Dog Complex."

43. Friedman, *Analyzing Freud*, 31.

44. *Ibid.*

45. H. D. Letter to Bryher, March 15, 1933, in Friedman, *Analyzing Freud*, 96.

46. Reiser, "Topsy—Living and Dying."

47. Coren, "Foreword."

48. *Ibid.*

49. H. D. Letter to Conrad Aiken, August 26, 1933, in Friedman, *Analyzing Freud*, 371.

50. Friedman, *Analyzing Freud*, 33.

51. Fine, *Handbook on Animal-Assisted Therapy*, 173–174.

52. Parish-Plass, "Animal-Assisted Therapy with Children Suffering from Insecure Attachment Due to Abuse and Neglect."

53. Levinson, *Pet-Oriented Child Psychotherapy,* 42.

54. Levinson, "The Dog as a 'Co-Therapist.'"

55. *Ibid.*

56. Coren, "How Therapy Dogs Almost Never Came to Exist."

57. Glucksman, "The Dog's Role in the Analyst's Consulting Room."

58. Fine, *Handbook of Animal-Assisted Therapy,* 173–174.

Chapter 3

1. To foment is to treat with moist heat. According to Gill in *Nightingales,* 93, Nightingale boiled the water before treating the dog's paw. This would not have been current practice at that time, and few doctors would have thought this necessary. If this version of the story is true, young Florence was already a skilled clinician.

2. The version of the story of Florence Nightingale and Cap which the author has presented in this chapter integrates details and part of versions of the story of Cap as it appears in several different Nightingale biographies. The version that appears here is based on Bostridge, *Florence Nightingale,* 45–47; Cook, *The Life of Florence Nightingale,* Vol. 1, 27, 98, 632–643; Knowles Bolton, *Lives of Girls Who Became Famous,* 91–93, 281–285; Gill, *Nightingales,* 91–93; Tooley, *Life of Florence Nightingale,* 27; McDonald, *Florence Nightingale: An Introduction to Her Life and Family,* Vol. 1, 58–59; Alldridge, *Florence Nightingale,* 10–15 Alldridge, writing in *Florence Nightingale,* 10–15, reported that the story originally appeared in *Little Folks Magazine* and quoted it as written in that magazine. Giffard published his remembrance of the event in 1867: *Constance and Cap, The Shepherd's Dog.* Cook reminisced about the event's significance. Giffard reported that the event took place in 1836 when Florence was 16. In *Life of Florence Nightingale,* Cook (p. 638) stated that the Rev. J. T. Giffard wrote to Florence Nightingale and asked if she remembered the Cap incident 22 years earlier. Cook further noted on p. 632 that the story was published with Nightingale's knowledge. Cap's treatment appeared to have saved his life from hanging. However, Bostridge noted on p. 46 that Nightingale later mentioned in a letter that she saw Cap running about on three legs, suggesting that while he may have had a long life after Florence's intervention, his leg may have eventually not survived.

3. *Ibid.*

4. Bostridge, *Florence Nightingale: The Making of an Icon,* xxii.

5. *Ibid.,* 46.

6. *Ibid.,* xxii.

7. *Ibid.,* 37.

8. *Ibid.,* xxi.

9. Nightingale, *Notes on Nursing,* 100, footnote 32.

10. Multiple biographies, books, and letters exist about the life and accomplishments of Florence Nightingale. This chapter offers various perspectives on her life and accomplishments, with a focus on the early period of Nightingale's life, and relied on multiple sources for her biographical profiles. Readers who would like to read more about her life are referred to Bostridge, *Florence Nightingale: The Making of an Icon*; Cook, *The Life of Florence Nightingale,* Vols. 1 and 2; Gill, *Nightingales*; McDonald, *The Collected Works of Florence Nightingale* (all volumes); Smith, *Florence Nightingale 1820–1910* and *Florence Nightingale: Reputation and Power*; Strachey, *Eminent Victorians*; Small, *Florence Nightingale: Avenging Angel*; Dossey, *Florence Nightingale: Mystic, Visionary, Reformer*; and Nightingale's *Notes on Nursing* and *Notes on Hospitals.*

11. See Smith, *Florence Nightingale: Reputation and Power*; Small, *Florence Nightingale: Avenging Angel.*

12. Strachey, *Eminent Victorians,* 66.

13. *Ibid.,* 77.

14. Bostridge, *Florence Nightingale: The Making of an Icon,* Prologue.

15. Scovil, "The Love Story of Florence Nightingale."

16. Greg, *Why Are Women Redundant?*

17. McDonald, *Florence Nightingale at First Hand,* 120–129.

18. Small, *Florence Nightingale: Avenging Angel,* 7–8.

19. Smith, *Florence Nightingale 1820–1910,* 10.

20. Stark, "Introduction," 11–15.

21. Nightingale Museum, *Florence Nightingale Biography.*

22. Smith, *Florence Nightingale 1820–1910,* 42.

23. *Ibid.*

24. Strachey, *Eminent Victorians.*

25. Rankin, "Florence Nightingale: Of Myths and Maths."

26. McDonald, *Florence Nightingale: An Introduction to Her Life and Family,* 10.

27. Smith, *Florence Nightingale 1820–1910,* 13.

28. *Ibid.,* 124.

29. Small, *Florence Nightingale: Avenging Angel,* 14.

30. *Ibid.*

31. Strachey, *Eminent Victorians,* 70.

32. McDonald, *Florence Nightingale at First Hand,* Preface, 38, 93.

33. Smith, *Florence Nightingale 1820–1910*, 41.
34. Jackson, *Dirty Old London*.
35. NPR, "A Dirty Old London," para. 13.
36. Nightingale Museum, *Florence Nightingale Biography*.
37. Nightingale, *Notes on Hospitals*, 59.
38. *Ibid.*, 64.
39. Smith, *Florence Nightingale: Reputation and Power*.
40. Nightingale, *Notes on Nursing*, 62.
41. *Ibid.*, 82.
42. McDonald, *Florence Nightingale at First Hand*, Preface, 38.
43. Bostridge, *Florence Nightingale: The Making of an Icon*, xxii.
44. McDonald, *Florence Nightingale at First Hand*, 3.
45. *Ibid.*, 68.
46. Gill, *Nightingales*, 92.
47. Alldridge, *Florence Nightingale*, 11.
48. Farmcollie.com. Retrieved September 15, 2017.
49. Dalton, "Farm Dogs."
50. Wright, "In Victorian England, a sheep wasn't just a sheep."
51. Dossey, "Florence Nightingale: Mystic, Visionary, Healer."
52. Bostridge, *Florence Nightingale: The Making of an Icon*, 46.
53. McDonald, *Florence Nightingale at First Hand*, 157. Also, chapter 1 notes that "Nightingale's recollection of conversion is in a letter of 1895 to Maude Verney, 8:927; Jacob Abbott, *The Corner Stone; Or, a Familiar Illustration of the Principles of Christian Truth* (London: T. Ward 1834)."
54. Cook, *The Life of Florence Nightingale*, Vol. 1, 1103.
55. Smith, *Florence Nightingale 1820–1910*, 13.
56. Dossey, "Florence Nightingale: Mystic, Visionary, Healer."
57. *Ibid.*
58. Underhill, *Practical Mysticism*, 102.
59. Dossey, "Florence Nightingale: Mystic, Visionary, Healer."
60. Coren, *Pawprints of History*, 11–14.
61. *Ibid.*, 1.
62. Coren, *Pawprints of History*, chapter 2 endnote.
63. Coren, "Florence Nightingale: The Dog and the Dream."
64. Beck, "The Five Secrets of Storytelling for Social Change."
65. Narrative medicine is a medical approach that recognizes the power of storytelling and utilizes personal narratives in clinical practice, research, and education as a way to promote healing. For more information, see http://sps.columbia.edu/narrative-medicine.
66. Norman, "Americans Rate Healthcare Providers High on Honesty, Ethics."
67. Coren, *Pawprints of History*, 291.
68. Rosenfeld, "Counterfactual Canines."
69. Bostridge, *Florence Nightingale: The Making of an Icon*, 46–47.
70. Pomerance, "Pets and Spirituality."
71. Anderson and Anderson, *Angel Dogs*, 10–11.
72. Bostridge, *Florence Nightingale*, Prologue.

Chapter 4

1. New York City Parks, "Central Park: Balto."
2. Seward Park Conservatory, "Togo."
3. Salisbury and Salisbury, *The Cruelest Miles*, 36.
4. Stokes, "The Race for Life," 273.
5. The highlights of the serum run to save Nome presented in this chapter are based on accounts of the race by several primary and secondary sources. Salisbury and Salisbury provided a comprehensive source for details of the run and the dog teams in their 2005 book, *The Cruelest Miles*. Additional material in this chapter is based on Ungermann's account of the run in his book *The Race to Nome*, originally published in 1963 with an updated edition in 2014. Another source was Leonhard Seppala's biography, *Seppala: Alaska Sled Dog Driver*, written by his friend and partner Elizabeth Ricker. Ricker's book includes Seppala's firsthand accounts of the run and background about his dogs, especially his relationship with Togo. An additional source was the 2003 book about the nurses of Alaska and the nurses who worked with Curtis Welch in *With a Dauntless Spirit: Alaska Nursing in Dog-Team Days*, edited by Effie Graham, Jackie Pflaum, and Elfrida Nord. Dr. Curtis Welch's letter, "The Diphtheria Epidemic at Nome," in the 1925 issue of the *Journal of the American Medical Association* provided a firsthand account by the doctor of his experience in diagnosing the disease and actions to prevent its spread. Information about Balto and the run was obtained from the Cleveland Museum of Natural History's brochure, *Balto and the Legacy of the Serum Run*, and Houdek, "The Serum Run of 1925." Additional sources for the chapter were journal and newspaper articles.
6. Albrecht, "Public Health in Alaska," 694–698.
7. Graham, Pflaum, and Nord, *With a Dauntless Spirit*, 13.
8. Stokes, "The Race for Life," 272.
9. Moyer, "Dog vs. Airplane," 2.

10. Aboul-Enein, Puddy, and Bowser, "The 1925 Diphtheria Antitoxin Run to Nome."

11. Graham, Pflaum, and Nord, *With a Dauntless Spirit*, 13.

12. *Ibid.*, 140.

13. *Ibid.*, 29.

14. Albrecht, "Public Health in Alaska," 694–700.

15. *Ibid.*, 695.

16. Parran and the Alaska Health Survey Team, *Alaska's Health: A Survey Report*.

17. Graham, Pflaum, and Nord, *With a Dauntless Spirit*, 3.

18. *Ibid.*, 33.

19. Stokes, "The Race for Life," 111.

20. Graham, Pflaum, and Nord, *With a Dauntless Spirit*, 21.

21. Kansas Historical Society, "Emily Morgan."

22. Ungermann, *The Race to Nome*, 127–132.

23. Museum of Healthcare at Kingston, "Diphtheria"; Centers for Disease Control and Prevention, "Iditarod."

24. *Ibid.*

25. Centers for Disease Control and Prevention, "About Diphtheria."

26. Centers for Disease Control and Prevention, "Iditarod."

27. *Ibid.*

28. *Ibid.*

29. Albrecht, "Public Health in Alaska," 697.

30. Alaska Humanities Forum, "Health and Medicine."

31. *Ibid.*

32. Salisbury and Salisbury, *The Cruelest Miles*, 39.

33. Welch, "The Diphtheria Epidemic at Nome."

34. Salisbury and Salisbury, *The Cruelest Mile*, 42.

35. Stokes, "The Race for Life," 273; Welch, "The Diphtheria Epidemic at Nome."

36. Scheindlin, "The Drug that Launched a Thousand Sleds"; Welch, "The Diphtheria Epidemic at Nome."

37. Ungermann, *The Race to Nome*, 235.

38. Salisbury and Salisbury, *The Cruelest Miles*, 126.

39. *Ibid.*, 158.

40. Stokes, "The Race for Life," 275.

41. Houdek, "The Serum Run of 1925."

42. Salisbury and Salisbury, *The Cruelest Miles*, 61.

43. Bragg, "Leonhard Seppala."

44. *Ibid.*

45. Ricker, *Seppala: Alaska Sled Dog Driver*, Foreword.

46. *Ibid.*, 283.

47. *Ibid.*, 284–285.

48. *Ibid.*, 284.

49. *Ibid.*

50. *Ibid.*

51. *Ibid.*, 284–288.

52. *Ibid.*, 283–285.

53. Salisbury and Salisbury, *The Cruelest Miles*, 159.

54. Ungermann, *The Race to Nome*, 939.

55. *Ibid.*

56. *Ibid.*, 280; Salisbury and Salisbury, *The Cruelest Miles*, 159.

57. Ungermann, *The Race to Nome*, 1021.

58. Ricker, *Seppala: Alaska Sled Dog Driver*, 295.

59. *Ibid.*, 281.

60. Aboul-Encin, Puddy, and Bowser, "The 1925 Diphtheria Antitoxin Run to Nome." Dunham, "Emily's Mission."

61. *Ibid.*

62. National Archives, Record Group 90.

63. Wilson, "The Serum Dash to Nome."

64. Coppock, "The Race to Save Nome."

65. Stokes, "The Race for Life," 273.

66. Moyer, "Dog vs. Airplane," 38–44.

67. Cleveland Museum of Natural History, *Balto and the Legacy of the Serum Run*.

68. *Ibid.*

69. Dunham, "Emily's Mission"; Kansas Historical Society, "Emily Morgan"; Alaska Women's Hall of Fame, "Emily Morgan."

70. Stokes, "The Race for Life," 272–275.

71. *Ibid.*; Cleveland Museum of Natural History, *Balto and the Legacy of the Serum Run*.

72. Ungermann, *The Race to Nome*, 1226.

73. Ricker, *Seppala: Alaska Sled Dog Driver*, 294–295.

74. *Ibid.*, 294–295.

75. *Ibid.*, 295.

76. Bragg, "Leonhard Seppala."

77. *Ibid.*

78. Salisbury and Salisbury, *The Cruelest Miles*, 259.

79. Welch, "The Diphtheria Epidemic at Nome."

80. Aboul-Encin, Puddy, and Bowser, "The 1925 Diphtheria Antitoxin Run to Nome."

81. *Ibid.*

82. Ungermann, *The Race to Nome*, 1206.

83. Stokes, "The Race for Life," 272–275.

84. Centers for Disease Control and Prevention, "Iditarod."

85. *Ibid.*

86. Ungermann, *The Race to Nome*, 1209.

87. Centers for Disease Control and Prevention, "Iditarod."

88. *Ibid.*

89. Alaska Department of Health and Human Services, "I Did It By TWO!" Campaign."

90. Alaska Humanities Forum, "Health and Medicine."

91. Alaska Department of Health and Human Services, "I Did It By TWO!" Campaign."
92. Gustkey, "The Iditarod."
93. Kuhl, "Human-Sled Dog Relationships."

Chapter 5

1. Clark and Frank, *First Lady of the Seeing Eye*, 39.
2. *Ibid.*, 39.
3. *Ibid.*, 40.
4. *Ibid.*, 39.
5. Putnam, *Love in the Lead*, 47.
6. Swanbeck, *Images of America*, 48.
7. Putnam, *Love in the Lead*, 48–50.
8. Morris Frank's memoir, *First Lady of the Seeing Eye*, cowritten with Blake Clark in 1957, was a major source for this chapter and provided Frank's detailed first-hand account of meeting Buddy and their work together. Peter Putnam, a historian who was also blind, provided a comprehensive history of the Seeing Eye organization history in his book, *Love in the Lead*. Putnam described the experience of working with a guide dog. Miriam Ascarelli's book, *Independent Vision*, provided information on Dorothy Harrison Eustis and the story of the Seeing Eye. The Seeing Eye Inc. provided a comprehensive source of information about guide dogs and its organizational history on its website.
9. The Seeing Eye, "History."
10. *Ibid.*
11. Eustis, "The Seeing Eye."
12. Clark and Frank, *First Lady of the Seeing Eye*, 15.
13. *Ibid.*, 15.
14. *Ibid.*, 16; Frank, Letter to Miss Dorothy Harrison Eustis, November 9, 1927.
15. *Ibid.*, 18.
16. *Ibid.*, 19.
17. *Ibid.*, 16.
18. The Seeing Eye, "About Vision Loss." For information on blindness and living with vision loss, see the websites of The Seeing Eye Inc. (http://www.seeingeye.org/knowledge-center/about-vision-loss.html), the American Federation for the Blind (https://www.afb.org/default.aspx), and the Centers for Disease Control and Prevention (https://www.cdc.gov/healthcommunication/toolstemplates/entertainmented/tips/Blindness.html).
19. Vanderbilt, "Through Buddy's Eyes."
20. Dickens, *American Notes*, chapter 3.
21. Putnam, *Love in the Lead*, 28.
22. *Ibid.*, 28–29.
23. *Ibid.*, 16.
24. Craigon et al., "She's a Dog at the End of the Day." Note that only dogs trained by The Seeing Eye, Inc., of Morristown, NJ, are properly called Seeing Eye˙ dogs. The Seeing Eye is a registered trademark. The generic term for dogs trained by other schools is "guide dog."
25. Ascarelli, *Independent Vision*, 37.
26. International Guide Dog Federation, "History of Guide Dogs."
27. Putnam, *Love in the Lead*, 10. German shepherds would later be used in World War II by the Allied and Axis forces as military dogs.
28. Swanbeck, *Images of America*, 10.
29. Ascarelli, *Independent Vision*, 37.
30. Putman, *Love in the Lead*, 12–13.
31. Treaster, "Elliott Humphrey."
32. Humphrey and Warner, *Working Dogs*.
33. Putnam, *Love in the Lead*, 17.
34. Scientific American, "German Shepherd Dogs."
35. Putman, *Love in the Lead*, 13–15.
36. *Ibid.*, 15.
37. *Ibid.*, 18.
38. Eustis, "The Seeing Eye."
39. Putnam, *Love in the Lead*, 25.
40. *Ibid.*, 39. See also Clark and Frank, *First Lady of the Seeing Eye*, 22–23.
41. Clark and Frank, *First Lady of the Seeing Eye*, 23.
42. *Ibid.*
43. Putnam, *Love in the Lead*, 16.
44. O'Toole, *Miller-Keane Encyclopedia & Dictionary*.
45. Swanbeck, *Images of America*, 65.
46. *Ibid.*
47. Ascarelli, *Independent Vision*, 37.
48. Swanbeck, *Images of America*, 56.
49. *Ibid.*, 54.
50. *Ibid.*, 55.
51. The Seeing Eye, "Frequently Asked Questions"; Swanbeck, *Images of America*, 54.
52. The Seeing Eye, "Frequently Asked Questions."
53. Swanbeck, *Images of America*, 62.
54. Clark and Frank, *First Lady of the Seeing Eye*, 28.
55. *Ibid.*
56. *Ibid.*, 88–89.
57. Clark and Frank, *First Lady of the Seeing Eye*, 79–80.
58. *Ibid.*, 92–93.
59. *Ibid.*, 109.
60. *Ibid.*, 133–135.
61. Clark and Frank, *First Lady of the Seeing Eye*, 149–150.
62. International Guide Dog Federation, "History of Guide Dogs."
63. Vanderbilt, "Through Buddy's Eyes."
64. *Ibid.*
65. The Seeing Eye website, www.seeingeye.org.

66. *Ibid.*

67. *Ibid.*

68. Swanbeck, *Images of America*, 49–51.

69. Lash, *Helen and Teacher*, 496–498.

70. Ensminger, *Service and Therapy Dogs in American Society,* 9.

71. Long, "May 16, 1938 Through Buddy's Eyes."

72. Ensminger, *Service and Therapy Dogs in American Society,* 48.

73. For a more detailed discussion of law and science as related to skilled dogs, access rights, and access and regulatory issues for service and therapy animals, see Ensminger, *Service and Therapy Dogs in American Society.*

74. U.S. Department of Justice, "ADA Requirements: Service Animals."

75. Bray et al., "Effects of Maternal Investment."

76. According to Merriam-Webster.com, *helicopter parent* is a term used to refer to a parent who is overly involved in the life of his or her child. It describes a parent "hovering" over his or her child like a helicopter.

77. Bray et al., "Effects of maternal investment."

78. *Ibid.*

79. Lloyd et al., "An Investigation of the Complexities of Successful and Unsuccessful Guide Dog Matching and Partnerships."

80. *Ibid.*

81. Nicholson et al., "Distress Arising from the End of a Guide Dog Partnership."

82. The Seeing Eye, *Annual Report 2016.*

83. Craigon et al., "She's a Dog at the End of the Day."

84. The Seeing Eye, "By the Numbers."

85. American Printing House for the Blind, "Morris Frank."

86. Clark and Frank, *First Lady of the Seeing Eye,* 156.

Chapter 6

1. Levinson, "The Dog as Cotherapist," 60; Levinson, *Pet-Oriented Child Psychotherapy,* 37–38.

2. *Ibid.*, 38.

3. *Ibid.*, 43.

4. *Ibid.*, 38.

5. Levinson provided a first-hand account of the story of Jingles in his book *Pet-Oriented Child Psychotherapy*, p. 43. Levinson also discussed his experience with Jingles as a pioneer in child psychotherapy in his paper "The Dog as a 'Co-Therapist'" in the journal *Mental Hygiene.* He discussed his experience with Jingles in his other papers and books. In his book, *Pet-Oriented Child Psychotherapy* (p. 37), he explained that Jingles played a leading role in his insight about dogs in psychotherapy. For more about his work with Jingles, see also Levinson, *Pets and Human Development,* and Levinson, "Pets: A Special Technique." The story of Jingles also appears in several other sources, including Chandler, "Animal-Assisted Therapy in Counseling," 23, and Coren, "Foreword."

6. Chandler, "Animal-Assisted Therapy in Counseling," 30.

7. Mallon, "Preface"; Levinson, *Pet-Oriented Child Psychotherapy*, 2nd ed., 37.

8. Searles, *The Nonhuman Environment.*

9. Rogers, "Psychotherapy Today or Where Do We Go from Here?"

10. Mallon, "Preface," x.

11. Coren, "How Therapy Dogs Almost Never Came to Exist."

12. *Ibid.*

13. Coren, "Foreword."

14. Levinson, *Pets and Human Development*, 154; Levinson, *Pet-Oriented Child Psychotherapy*, 43; Mallon, "Preface," xi.

15. Levinson, "The Dog as a 'Co-Therapist.'"

16. Levinson, "Pets: A Special Technique," 243.

17. Levinson, "Pets: A Special Technique," 248; Mallon, "Preface," xi.

18. Levinson, *Pet-Oriented Child Psychotherapy*, 37.

19. Levinson, "The Dog as a 'Co-Therapist.'"

20. Mallon, "Preface."

21. *Ibid.*

22. Levinson, "The Dog as a 'Co-Therapist,'" 60.

23. Levinson, "Pets: A Special Technique," 376.

24. Levinson, "The Dog as a 'Co-Therapist,'" 61.

25. *Ibid.*

26. Melson, *Why the Wild Things Are,* 108–111, 119–123.

27. Mallon, "Preface," ix.

28. Levinson, "The Dog as a 'Co-Therapist,'" "Pets: A Special Technique," *Pet-Oriented Child Psychotherapy.*

29. Levinson, "The Dog as a 'Co-Therapist.'"

30. *Ibid.*, 65.

31. *Ibid.*

32. Melson, *Why the Wild Things Are,* 108–111, 119–123.

33. Levinson, "The Dog as a 'Co-Therapist,'" 61.

34. Levinson, "Pets: A Special Technique," 381.

35. Levinson, "The Dog as a 'Co-Therapist,'" 64.

36. Levinson, "Pets: A Special Technique."

37. Levinson, *Pet-Oriented Child Psychotherapy*, 376–382.

38. *Ibid.*

39. Serpell, "Animal Companions and Human Well-Being."

40. Chandler, *Animal-Assisted Therapy in Counseling.*

41. Jones, *Lunacy, Law, and Conscience,* 59–61.

42. Chandler, *Animal-Assisted Therapy in Counseling,* 19.

43. Parshall, "Research and Reflection," 47.

44. D'Amore, "Introduction."

45. *Ibid.*

46. Chandler, *Animal-Assisted Therapy in Counseling,* 22; Blum and Fee, "Howard A. Rusk."

47. Chandler, *Animal-Assisted Therapy in Counseling,* 22.

48. Draper, Gerber, and Layng, "Defining the Role of Pet Animals."

49. Levinson, *Pet-Oriented Child Psychotherapy,* 39.

50. Levinson, "Pets: A Special Technique," 382.

51. Levinson, "The Future of Research."

52. *Ibid.*

53. *Ibid.,* 283.

54. Levinson, "The Future of Research."

55. *Ibid.,* 291–292.

56. Levinson, *Pet-Oriented Child Psychotherapy,* 169.

57. Mallon, "Utilization of Animals as Therapeutic Adjuncts," 53.

58. Goddard and Gilmer, "The Role and Impact of Animals with Pediatric Patients."

59. *Ibid.*

60. *Ibid.,* 37.

61. Levinson, *Pet-Oriented Child Psychotherapy.*

Chapter 7

1. Fike, Najera, and Dougherty, "Occupational Therapists as Dog Handlers."

2. Krol, "Training the Combat and Operational Stress Control Dog."

3. Smith-Forbes et al., "Combat Operational Stress Control in Iraq and Afghanistan." Several articles in the journal *U.S. Army Medical Department Journal,* April-June 2012 issue provided primary and secondary source material for this chapter. This journal is a collection of articles rich with details about animal-assisted therapy in military medicine, the COSC dogs and the therapy dogs' role in the military and may be interesting to readers who would like to explore the role of animal assisted therapy in the military.

4. Chumley, "Historical Perspectives of the Human-Animal Bond."

5. Smith-Forbes et al., "Combat Operational Stress Control in Iraq and Afghanistan."

6. Fike, Najera, and Dougherty, "Occupational Therapists as Dog Handlers."

7. Rumayor and Thrasher, "Reflections on Recent Research," 110.

8. Kaplan, "Dogs Bring Relief to Soldiers."

9. Fike, Najera, and Dougherty, "Occupational Therapists as Dog Handlers," 53.

10. *Ibid.,* 54.

11. Kaplan, " Dogs Bring Relief to Soldiers."

12. Gregg, "Crossing the Berm."

13. *Ibid.*

14. Serpell, "Animal-Assisted Interventions in Historical Perspective."

15. Frankel, *War Dogs,* 269.

16. *Ibid.,* chapter 59; Libby, *Reporting for Duty,* chapter 4.

17. Libby, *Reporting for Duty,* chapter 4.

18. *Ibid.*

19. Wynne, *Yorkie Doodle Dandy,* 214–406.

20. Frankel, "Dogs at War."

21. Levinson, "The Dog as a 'Co-Therapist.'"

22. Chumley, "Historical Perspectives of the Human-Animal Bond."

23. Knisely et al., "Research on Benefits of Canine-Assisted Therapy"; O'Haire et al., "Animal-Assisted Intervention for Trauma."

24. Chapter 8 discusses the role of modern therapy dogs in various settings.

25. America's VetDogs, "About America's VetDogs."

26. Chapter 8 describes differences between therapy dogs, service dogs and their rights of access.

27. Krol, "Training the Combat and Operational Stress Control Dog."

28. Headquarters, Department of the Army, *Field Manual 4-02.51*; Smith-Forbes et al., "Combat Operational Stress Control in Iraq and Afghanistan."

29. Headquarters, Department of the Army, *Field Manual 4-02.51.*

30. Ritchie and Amaker, "Canine-Assisted Therapy in Military Medicine."

31. American Occupational Therapy Association, "Standards of Practice."

32. U.S. Army, "Careers & Jobs: Occupational Therapist."

33. Smith-Forbes et al., "Combat Operational Stress Control in Iraq and Afghanistan."

34. *Ibid.*

35. Krol, "Training the Combat and Operational Stress Control Dog," 46–47.

36. Mayo Health, "Mental Health: Overcoming the Stigma of Mental Illness."

37. Dingfelder, "The Military's War on Stigma."

38. Regier et al., "The De Facto U.S. Mental and Addictive Disorders Service System";

Department of Health and Human Services, *Mental Health: A Report of the Surgeon General*, 8.

39. National Alliance on Mental Illness, "Stigma*free*."

40. Corrigan, Druss, and Perlick, "The Impact of Mental Illness Stigma."

41. American Psychological Association, "Psychological Needs of Military Personnel"; Corrigan, Druss, and Perlick, "The Impact of Mental Illness Stigma."

42. Department of Health and Human Services, *Mental Health: A Report of the Surgeon General.*

43. *Ibid.*

44. *Ibid.*, 9.

45. Dingfelder, "The Military's War on Stigma."

46. Acosta et al., *Mental Health Stigma in the Military.*

47. *Ibid.*

48. *Ibid.*

49. Krol, "Training the Combat and Operational Stress Control Dog."

50. Gregg, "Crossing the Berm."

51. *Ibid.*

52. Krol, "Training the Combat and Operational Stress Control Dog."

53. *Ibid.*

54. Frenkel, *War Dogs*, chapter 57.

55. Ritchie and Amaker, "Canine-Assisted Therapy in Military Medicine."

56. *Ibid.*

57. Rumayor and Thrasher, "Reflections on Recent Research," 110; Baldor, "Therapy Dogs Help Treat Soldiers"; Cunningham, "Top Dogs," Amison, "Therapy Dog Brightens Lives"; Pet Partners, "Major Rumayor and Lexy."

58. Rumayor and Thrasher, "Reflections on Recent Research," 109–110.

59. Rumayor and Thrasher, "Reflections on Recent Research"; Ritchie and Amaker, "Canine-Assisted Therapy in Military Medicine."

Chapter 8

1. Pet Partners, "About Us."

2. Marr et al., "Animal-Assisted Therapy in Psychiatric Rehabilitation."

3. Carolyn Marr, email communication to author, June 8, 2018.

4. Pet Partners Greater Dallas, "What We Do."

5. Texas Health Resources, "Some Hospital Volunteers are a Breed Apart."

6. Susan Schultz, Personal communication, January 5, 2018; Carolyn Marr, email communication, June 8, 2018.

7. Carolyn Marr, email communication, June 8, 2018.

8. Susan Schultz, personal communication, January 5, 2018; Carolyn Marr, email communication, June 8, 2018.

9. Carolyn Marr, email communication, June 8, 2018.

10. Gloria Dei Garland, "Creature Care."

11. Carolyn Marr, email communication, June 8, 2018.

12. *Ibid.*

13. American Kennel Club, "Therapy Dog Programs."

14. López-Cepero Borrego et al., "Animal-Assisted Interventions."

15. Fine and Beck, "Understanding Our Kinship with Animals," 3–15.

16. Chandler, *Animal-Assisted Therapy in Counseling*, 29; Kamioka et al., "Effectiveness of Animal-Assisted Therapy"; Nimer and Lundahl, "Animal-Assisted Therapy: A Meta-Analysis."

17. Turner, "The Role of Ethology."

18. Pet Partners, "The Pet Partners Story." McCullough, Bill, "Letter From the Founder." Excerpts from the Milestones in History of Delta Society and Pet Partners in "A Letter from the Founder" and information on history of Pet Partners are used with permission of Pet Partners.

19. *Ibid.*

20. Williams, "From the Medical Perspective."

21. *Ibid.*

22. Pet Partners, "Financial Information."

23. Therapy Dogs International, Homepage; Alliance of Therapy Dogs, Homepage; Ensminger, *Service and Therapy Dogs in American Society: Science, Law and the Evolution of Canine Caregivers.*

24. Chandler, *Animal-Assisted Therapy in Counseling*, 30.

25. American Psychological Association, "Human-Animal Interaction."

26. *Ibid.* Section 17 also addresses education programs and violence prevention and the link between animal abuse and family, juvenile, and community violence.

27. Chandler, *Animal-Assisted Therapy in Counseling*, 30; American Counseling Association, "Interest Networks."

28. McCullough et al., "The Use of Dogs."

29. Kruger and Serpell, "Animal-Assisted Interventions in Mental Health."

30. For a detailed discussion on more theoretical frameworks of the human-animal bond, see Kruger and Serpell, "Animal-Assisted Interventions in Mental Health."

31. Kruger and Serpell, "Animal-Assisted Interventions in Mental Health."

32. *Ibid.*; Kahn, "Developmental Psychol-

ogy and the Biophilia Hypothesis"; Wilson, *Biophilia*.

33. Fine and Beck, "Understanding Our Kinship with Animals," 7; Kahn, "Developmental Psychology and the Biophilia Hypothesis."

34. Bowlby, *Attachment and Loss*.

35. Kruger and Serpell, "Animal-Assisted Interventions in Mental Health."

36. Beck and Katcher, "A New Look at Pet-Facilitated Therapy."

37. *Ibid.*, 415.

38. *Ibid.*

39. Borrego et al., "Animal-Assisted Interventions."

40. Barker et al., "Benefits of Interacting with Companion Animals"; Wilkes et al., "Pet Therapy: Implications for Good Health"; Chandler, *Animal-Assisted Therapy in Counseling*, 4–5; Fine et al., "Forward Thinking"; Pet Partners, "Benefits of the Human-Animal Bond."

41. The author has discussed a few examples of AAI and AAT research studies in the chapter. For more studies see Banks and Banks, "The Effects of Animal-Assisted Therapy on Loneliness"; Barba, "The Positive Influence of Animals"; Barker, Knisely, Schubert, Green, and Ameringer, "The Effect of an Animal-Assisted Intervention on Anxiety and Pain"; Beck and Katcher, "A New Look at Pet-Facilitated Therapy"; Binfet, "The Effects of Group-Administered Canine Therapy"; Braun et al., "Animal-Assisted Therapy as a Pain Relief Intervention"; Burke and Iannuzzi, "Animal-Assisted Therapy for Children and Adolescents with Autism Spectrum Disorders"; Calvo et al., "Animal Assisted Therapy (AAT) Program as a Useful Adjunct to Conventional Psychosocial Rehabilitation"; Cole et al., "Animal-Assisted Therapy in Patients Hospitalized with Heart Failure"; Creagan, Bauer, Thomley, and Borg, "Animal-Assisted Therapy at Mayo Clinic"; Germain, Wilkie, Milbourne, and Theule, "Animal-Assisted Psychotherapy and Trauma"; Ginex et al., "Animal-Facilitated Therapy Program"; Holcomb and Meacham, "Effectiveness of an Animal-Assisted Therapy Program"; Hundley, "Pet Project"; Hunt and Chizkov, "Are Therapy Dogs Like Xanax?"; Knisley et al., "Research on Benefits of Canine-Assisted Therapy"; Lundqvist, Carlsson, Sjödahl, Theodorsson, and Levin, "Patient Benefit of Dog-Assisted Interventions"; Maujean, Pepping, and Kendall, "A Systematic Review of Randomized Controlled Trials of Animal-Assisted Therapy"; McCullough et al., "Measuring the Effects of an Animal-Assisted Intervention"; McCullough et al., "Physiological and Behavioral Effects of Animal-Assisted Interventions"; Nepps et al., "Animal-Assisted Activity"; Nimer and Lundahl, "Animal-Assisted Therapy: A Meta-Analysis"; O'Haire, "Animal-Assisted Intervention for Autism Spectrum Disorder"; O'Haire, Guérin, and Kirkham, "Animal-Assisted Intervention for Trauma"; White et al., "Animal-Assisted Therapy and Counseling Support"; Wood, Ohlsen, Thompson, Hulin, and Knowles, "The Feasibility of Brief Dog-Assisted Therapy."

42. Maujean, Pepping, and Kendall, "A Systematic Review of Randomized Controlled Trials of Animal-Assisted Therapy"; McCune et al., "Strengthening the Foundation of Human-Animal Interaction Research"; Lundqvist, Carlsson, Sjödahl, Theodorsson, and Levin, "Patient Benefit of Dog-Assisted Interventions"; Hosey and Melfi, "Human-Animal Interactions, Relationships and Bonds"; Rumayor and Thrasher, "Reflections on Recent Research."

43. A meta-analysis is a quantitative, formal, statistical analysis used to systematically assess previous research studies to derive conclusions about that body of research. Outcomes from a meta-analysis may include a more precise estimate of the effect of treatment or risk factor for disease, or other outcomes, than any individual study contributing to the pooled analysis. See Haidich, "Meta-Analysis in Medical Research."

44. Nimer and Lundahl, "Animal-Assisted Therapy: A Meta-Analysis."

45. *Ibid.*

46. Cole et al., "Animal-Assisted Therapy in Patients Hospitalized with Heart Failure."

47. Nepps et al., "Animal-Assisted Activity: Effects of a Complementary Intervention Program." https://www.ncbi.nlm.nih.gov/pubmed/?term=Stewart CN%5BAuthor%5D&cauthor=true&cauthor_uid=24789913

48. Barker and Dawson, "The Effects of Animal-Assisted Therapy on Anxiety Ratings."

49. Banks and Banks, "The Effects of Animal-Assisted Therapy on Loneliness."

50. *Ibid.*

51. Cherniack and Cherniack, "The Benefit of Pets and Animal-Assisted Therapy."

52. Moretti et al., "Pet Therapy in Elderly Patients with Mental Illness."

53. O'Haire, Guérin, and Kirkham, "Animal-Assisted Intervention for Trauma."

54. Orlandi et al., "Pet Therapy Effects on Oncological Day Hospital Patients."

55. Gagnon et al., "Implementing a Hospital-Based Animal Therapy Program for Children with Cancer."

56. White et al., "Animal-Assisted Therapy and Counseling Support for Women with Breast Cancer."

57. Orlandi et al., "Pet Therapy Effects on Oncological Day Hospital Patients."

58. See studies available in the research sec-

tion of the Center for Human-Animal Interaction (https://chai.vcu.edu/research/): Barker
et al., "A Randomized Crossover Exploratory
Study"; Barker et al., "Therapy Dogs on Campus"; Knisely et al., "Research on Benefits of
Canine-Assisted Therapy"; Barker and Dawson, "The Effects of Animal-Assisted Therapy
on Anxiety Ratings"; Barker et al., "The Effect
of an Animal-Assisted Intervention on Anxiety
and Pain"; Barker and Barker, "The Human-
Canine Bond"; Wood et al., "The Feasibility of
Brief Dog-Assisted Therapy."

59. Barker et al., "Measuring Stress and Immune Response in Healthcare Professionals."

60. Rossetti et al., "Behavioral Health Staff's
Perceptions of Pet-Assisted Therapy."

61. Feldman, "The Power of the Pet Effect."

62. Miller et al., "An Examination of Changes
in Oxytocin Levels"; Odendaal and Meintjes,
"Neurophysiological Correlates of Affiliative
Behavior Between Humans and Dogs"; Oden-
daal, "Animal-Assisted Therapy—Magic or
Medicine?"; Pop et al., "Physiological Effects
of Human-Animal Positive Interaction in
Dogs"; Moretti et al., "Pet Therapy in Elderly
Patients with Mental Illness."

63. Human-Animal Bond Research Insti-
tute, "Research"; Odendaal and Meintjes,
"Neurophysiological Correlates of Affiliative
Behavior Between Humans and Dogs."

64. Stull, Hoffman, and Landers, "Health
Benefits and Risks of Pets in Nursing Homes."

65. Glenk, "Current Perspectives on Therapy Dog Welfare."

66. *Ibid.*

67. McCullough, "Physiological and Behavioral Effects of Animal-Assisted Interventions."

68. *Ibid.*

69. International Association of Human-
Animal Interaction Organizations, *The IA-
HAIO Definitions.*

70. Griffin et al., "Scientific Research on
Human-Animal Interaction."

71. Wilson and Barker, "Challenges in Designing Human-Animal Interaction Research."

72. Chur-Hansen et al., "Animal-Assisted
Interventions in Children's Hospitals."

73. *Ibid.*

74. Human-Animal Bond Research Institute, "Research."

75. HABRI Central, home page: https://
habricentral.org/.

76. International Association of Human-
Animal Interaction Organizations, *The IA-
HAIO Definitions.* Definitions are reprinted
here with permission of the International Association of Human-Animal Interaction Organizations.

77. *Ibid.*

78. *Ibid.*

79. *Ibid.*

80. *Ibid.*

81. Labelle, "Considering Pet Therapy?"

82. Pet Partners.org, "Terminology."

83. *Ibid.*

84. *Ibid.*

85. *Ibid.*

86. Pet Partners, "Terminology."

87. Schilp, "Rescued Husky Returns Favor
in Texas."

88. *Ibid.*

89. Fontenot, Email communication to author.

90. *Ibid.*

91. Coren, "Foreword."

92. VanFleet and Faa-Thompson, *Animal
Assisted Play Therapy,* 15–16.

93. *Ibid.*

94. Fine, *Handbook on Animal-Assisted
Therapy.*

95. Pet Partners, "Benefits of the Human-
Animal Bond."

96. Gammonley et al., *Animal-Assisted
Therapy: Therapeutic Interventions*; Howie,
"Sample Goals and Methods."

97. Chandler, *Animal-Assisted Therapy in
Counseling,* 197.

98. O'Callaghan and Chandler, "An Exploratory Study of Animal-Assisted Interventions Utilized by Mental Health Professionals."
For a discussion and description of AAT interventions and intentions, also see Chandler,
Animal-Assisted Therapy in Counseling, 139.

99. Chandler, *Animal-Assisted Therapy in
Counseling,* 197.

100. Chur-Hansen et al., "Animal-Assisted
Interventions in Children's Hospitals."

101. McCullough et al., *The Use of Dogs in
Hospital Settings.*

102. Murthy et al., "Animals in Healthcare
Facilities," 7.

103. McCullough et al., *The Use of Dogs in
Hospitals Settings*; Chur-Hansen et al., "*Animal-
Assisted Interventions in Children's Hospitals.*"
Infection Control Today, "Transmission-Pre-
vention Cleaning Procedure Prevents Therapy
Dogs Spreading MRSA to Children With Can-
cer."

104. Labelle, "Considering Pet Therapy?"

105. Linder, Siebens, Mueller, Gibbs, and
Freeman, "Animal-Assisted Interventions: A
National Survey."

106. *Ibid.*

107. Labelle, "Considering Pet Therapy?"

108. For a complete list of guidelines for
human and animal well-being in AAI and
animal-assisted activity, see International Association of Human-Animal Interaction Organizations, *The IAHAIO Definitions.*

109. International Association of Human-

Animal Interaction Organizations, *The IA-HAIO Definitions*, 7–9.

110. Murthy et al., "Animals in Healthcare Facilities." The Society for Healthcare Epidemiology of America (SHEA) Guidelines Committee comprising experts in infection control and prevention developed the recommendations based on available evidence, practical considerations, a survey of SHEA members, writing group opinion, and consideration of potential harm, where applicable.

111. "New Guidance for Animal Hospital Visits Released."

112. Lefebvre et al., "Guidelines for AAIs in Health Care Facilities."

113. American Veterinary Medical Association, "AVMA Animal Welfare Principles."

114. McCullough et al., *The Use of Dogs in Hospital Settings*, 5.

115. Rabinowitz, "Training Health Care Providers about the Human-Animal Bond.," See Chapter Nine for more information on *One Health*.

116. *Ibid.*

117. *Ibid.*

118. American Humane, "Press Release."

Chapter 9

1. Grandin and Johnson, "Animals in Translation," 7.

2. Campbell, *The Hero with a Thousand Faces*.

3. Langley et al., *The Improvement Guide*.

4. *Ibid.*, XXL.

5. Rogers, *Diffusion of Innovations*.

6. American Veterinary Medical Association, "Human-Animal Bond."

7. Fine, *Handbook on Animal-Assisted Therapy*, 4th ed., 358.

8. *Ibid.*, 371.

9. International Association of Human-Animal Interaction organizations, The IA-HAIO Definitions.

10. McCullough et al., "Physiological and Behavioral Effects."

11. Rugaas, *On Talking Terms with Dogs*; Gammonley et al., *Animal-Assisted Therapy: Therapeutic Interventions*.

12. For a discussion of calming signals in dogs see Rugaas, *On Talking Terms with Dogs*.

13. For a discussion of a "therapy dog bill of rights," see Howie, *Teaming with Your Therapy Dog*.

14. Brambell, *Report of the Technical Committee*.

15. American Society for the Prevention of Cruelty to Animals, "The Five Freedoms."

16. American Veterinary Medical Association, "Animal Welfare: What Is It?"

17. World Organization for Animal Health, "Animal Welfare."

18. Association of Shelter Veterinarians, "The Five Freedoms."

19. Mellor, "Moving Beyond the 'Five Freedoms.'"

20. Tedeschi, "The New Work of Intervention and Assistance Dogs."

21. *Ibid.*

22. International Association of Human-Animal Interaction Organizations, *The IA-HAIO Definitions*, 5–7.

23. Grandin and Johnson, *Animals in Translation*; Grandin and Johnson, "Animals Make Us Human"; Mousson and McCarthy, *When Elephants Weep*; Bekoff, *The Emotional Life of Animals*; Horowitz, *Inside of a Dog*.

24. Grandin and Johnson. *Animals in Translation*, 8.

25. King et al., "Executive Summary of the AVMA One Health Initiative Task Force Report."

26. Natterson-Horowitz and Bowers, *Zoobiquity*.

27. One Health Initiative, "About the One Health Initiative."

28. Centers for Disease Control and Prevention, "One Health Basics."

29. Centers for Disease Control and Prevention, "One Health Basics" and "One Health Initiative."

30. UC Davis, "One Health."

31. *Ibid.*

32. National Link Coalition, "What is the Link?"

33. *Ibid.*

34. *Ibid.*

Epilogue

1. Katz, *A Dog Year*.

2. This story previously appeared in a blog post on the author's blog at www.Jillschilp.com.

Glossary

1. American Psychological Association, "Dictionary of Psychology."

2. International Association of Human-Animal Interaction Organizations, *The IA-HAIO Definitions*.

3. *Ibid.*

4. *Ibid.*

5. *Ibid.*

6. *Ibid.*

7. The Seeing Eye, "About Vision Loss."

8. American Psychological Association, "Dictionary of Psychology."

9. *Ibid.*

10. *Ibid.*

11. Rogers, *Diffusion of Innovations.*

12. Centers for Disease Control and Prevention. "About Diphtheria."

13. Centers for Disease Control and Prevention. "Diphtheria."

14. Pet Partners, "Terminology."

15. *Ibid.*

16. Merriam Webster online: https://www.merriam-webster.com/dictionary/foment.

17. American Psychoanalytic Association, "Psychoanalytic Terms."

18. American Veterinary Medical Association, "Human-Animal Bond"; Pet Partners, "Terminology."

19. Centers for Disease Control and Prevention, "Immunization: The Basics."

20. Haidich, "Meta-Analysis in Medical Research."

21. Merriam Webster online: https://www.merriam-webster.com/dictionary/metaphor.

22. American Occupational Therapy Association, "Standards of Practice."

23. American Veterinary Medical Association, "One Health—It's All Connected."

24. International Association of Human-Animal Interaction Organizations, *The IAHAIO Definitions.*

25. American Psychological Association, "Dictionary of Psychology."

26. *Ibid.*

27. American Psychoanalytic Association, "Psychoanalytic Terms."

28. American Psychoanalytic Association, "Psychoanalytic Terms."

29. Mayo Clinic, "Mental Health: Overcoming the Stigma of Mental Illness."

30. National Link Coalition, "What is the Link?"

31. American Psychological Association, "Dictionary of Psychology."

32. Pet Partners, "Terminology."

33. American Psychological Association, "Dictionary of Psychology."

34. Tabers Medical Dictionary Online: https://www.tabers.com/tabersonline/view/Tabers-Dictionary/735812/all/triage?q=triage.

35. Centers for Disease Control and Prevention, "Diphtheria."

Bibliography

Aboul-Enein, Basil H., William C. Puddy, and Jacqueline E. Bowser. "The 1925 Diphtheria Antitoxin Run to Nome–Alaska: A Public Health Illustration of Human-Animal Collaboration." *Journal of the Medical Humanities* 2016. https://doi.org/10.1007/s10912-016-9428-y.

Acosta, Joie D., Amariah Becker, Jennifer L. Cerully, Michael P. Fisher, Laurie T. Martin, Raffaele Vardavas, Mary Ellen Slaughter, and Terry Schell. *Mental Health Stigma in the Military.* Santa Monica, CA: Rand Corporation, 2014. https://www.rand.org/content/dam/rand/pubs/research_reports/RR400/RR426/RAND_RR426.pdf.

Alaska Department of Health and Human Services. *"I Did It By TWO!" Campaign,* 2016.

Alaska Humanities Forum. "Chapter 4–21: Health and Medicine." In *Alaska's Heritage,* 2017. http://www.akhistorycourse.org/americas-territory/alaskas-heritage/chapter-4-21-health-and-medicine.

Alaska Women's Hall of Fame. "Emily Morgan." Accessed October 4, 2017. http://alaskawomenshalloffame.org/alumnae/name/emily-morgan/.

Albrecht, C. Earl. "Public Health in Alaska—United States Frontier." *American Journal of Public Health* 42 (1952): 694–98.

Alldridge, Lizzie. *Florence Nightingale, Frances Ridley Havergal, Catherine March, Mrs. Ranyard.* London: Cassel and Company, 1885.

Allen, Karen, Barbara E. Shykoff, and Joseph L. Izzo. "Pet Ownership, But Not ACE Inhibitor Therapy, Blunts Home Blood Pressure Responses to Mental Stress." *Hypertension* 38, no. 4 (2001): 815–20.

Alliance of Therapy Dogs. Home page. Accessed June 15, 2018. https://www.therapydogs.com.

"Ambulance Dogs." *The British Medical Journal* 2 (1910, December 10), 1589–90.

American Counseling Association. "Interest Networks." Accessed April 30, 2018. https://www.counseling.org/aca-community/aca-groups/interest-networks#Animal.

American Humane Association. "Press Release" Accessed October 14, 2018. https://www.americanhumane.org/press-release/dog-who-lost-nearly-all-four-legs-but-never-lost-hope-wins-top-title-of-american-hero-dog-at-the-2018-american-humane-hero-dog-awards/

American Humane Association. "Print and Post Five Freedoms." Accessed June 15, 2018. https://www.aspcapro.org/resource/print-and-post-five-freedoms.

American Kennel Club. "Therapy Dog Program." Accessed August 30, 2018. https://www.akc.org/products-services/training-programs/akc-therapy-dog-program/

American Occupational Therapy Association. "About Occupational Therapy." Accessed November 15, 2017. https://www.aota.org/About-Occupational-Therapy.aspx.

American Occupational Therapy Association. "Occupational Therapy Roles." *American Journal of Occupational Therapy* 47 (1993): 1087–99. doi: 10.5014/ajot.47.12.1087.

American Occupational Therapy Association. "Standards of Practice for Occupational Therapy." Revised 2010. https://www.aota.org/~/media/Corporate/Files/AboutAOTA/Core/Standards%20of%20Practice%20for%20Occupational%20Therapy%20FINAL.pdf.

American Occupational Therapy Association. "What Is Occupational Therapy?" Accessed November 15, 2017. https://www.aota.org/Conference-Events/OTMonth/what-is-OT.aspx.

American Printing House for the Blind. "Morris Frank." In Hall of Fame: Leaders and Legends of the Blindness Field. Accessed August 30, 2018. https://www.aph.org/hall/inductees/frank/

American Psychoanalytic Association. "Psychoanalytic Terms and Concepts Defined." Accessed August 3, 2017. http://www.apsa.org/content/psychoanalytic-terms-concepts-defined.

American Psychological Association. "Dictionary of Psychology." Accessed June 15, 2018. https://dictionary.apa.org/

American Psychological Association. "Human-Animal Interaction, Section 13 of Division 17 of the American Psychological Association." Accessed June 15, 2018. https://www.apa-hai.org/human-animal-interaction.

American Psychological Association. "Psychological Needs of Military Personnel and Their Families Are Increasing—Straining Military Health Care System, Reports APA Task Force," Press release, February 25, 2007. http://www.apa.org/news/press/releases/2007/02/military-health.aspx.

American Society for the Prevention of Cruelty to Animals. "The Five Freedoms" [flyer]. Accessed January 3, 2018. https://www.aspcapro.org/resource/print-and-post-five-freedoms.

American Veterinary Medical Association. "Animal Welfare: What Is It?" Accessed April 20, 2018. https://www.avma.org/KB/Resources/Reference/AnimalWelfare/Pages/what-is-animal-welfare.aspx.

American Veterinary Medical Association. "AVMA Animal Welfare Principles." Accessed December 26, 2017. https://www.avma.org/KB/Policies/Pages/AVMA-Animal-Welfare-Principles.aspx.

American Veterinary Medical Association. "Guidelines for Animal-Assisted Activity, Animal-Assisted Therapy and Resident Animal Programs." Revised 2006, Reaffirmed 2011. https://ebusiness.avma.org/files/productdownloads/guidelines_AAA.pdf.

American Veterinary Medical Association. "Human-Animal Bond." Accessed December 26, 2017. https://www.avma.org/kb/resources/reference/human-animal-bond/pages/human-animal-bond-avma.aspx.

American Veterinary Medical Association. "One Health—It's All Connected." Accessed May 4, 2018. https://www.avma.org/KB/Resources/Reference/Pages/One-Health.aspx.

American War Dog Association. War Dog History. Accessed July 11, 2017. http://www.uswardogs.org/war-dog-history/world-war-1/

Americans with Disabilities Act of 1990. Public Law 101–336. 108th Congress, 2nd session. July 26, 1990. http://library.clerk.house.gov/reference-files/PPL_101_336_Americans WithDisabilities.pdf.

America's VetDogs. "About America's Vet-Dogs." Accessed November 15, 2017. ttps://www.vetdogs.org/AV/About/AV/About_Us/about_us.aspx?hkey=6bcdc249-95bd-4a4b-ac70-7e13e500f95d.

Amison, Mary-Dale. "Therapy Dog Brightens Lives." Accessed November 15, 2017. https://www.defense.gov/News/Article/Article/1230585/therapy-dog-brightens-lives

Anderson, Linda, and Allen Anderson. Angel Dogs: Divine Messengers of Love. Novato, CA: New World Library, 2005.

Andreasen, Gena Tiffany Stella, Megan Wilkison, Christy Szczech Moser, Allison Hoelzel, and Laura Hendricks. "Animal-Assisted Therapy and Occupational Therapy." Journal of Occupational Therapy, Schools, & Early Intervention 10, no. 1 (2017): 1–17. doi:10.1080/19411243.2017.1287519.

Arkow, Phil. Animal-Assisted Therapy and Activities: A Study, Resource Guide and Bibliography for the Use of Companion Animals in Selected Therapies, 10th ed. Stratford, NJ: P. Arkow, 2011.

Ascarelli, Miriam. Independent Vision: Dorothy Harrison Eustis and the Story of the Seeing Eye. West Lafayette, IN: Purdue University Press, 2010.

Ascione, Frank R. Children and Animals: Exploring the Roots of Kindness and Cruelty. West Lafayette, IN: Purdue University Press, 2005.

Ascione, Frank R. "Children Who Are Cruel to Animals: A Review of Research and Implications for Developmental Psychopathology." Anthrozoös 6 (1993): 226–47.

Assistance Dogs International. "Standards." Accessed November 15, 2017. http://www.assistancedogsinternational.org/standards/.

Association of Shelter Veterinarians. "The Five Freedoms." Accessed January 6, 2018. http://www.sheltervet.org/five-freedoms.

Audrestch, Hilary M., Chantelle T. Whelan, David Grice, Lucy Asher, Gary England, and Sarah L Freeman. "Recognizing the Value of Assistance Dogs in Society." Disability and Health Journal 8, no. 4 (2015): 469–74. http://dx.doi.org/10.1016/j.dhjo.2015.07.001.

Bacon, B. L., and J. J. Staudenmeier. "A Historical Overview of Combat Stress Control Units of the U.S. Army." Military Medicine 168 (2003): 689–93.

Baldor, Lolita C. "Therapy Dogs Help Treat Soldiers." Albuquerque Journal, June 20, 2014. https://www.abqjournal.com/418090/therapy-dogs-help-treat-soldiers.html.

Banks, Marian R., and William A. Banks. "The Effects of Animal-Assisted Therapy on

Loneliness in an Elderly Population in Long-Term Care Facilities." *The Journals of Gerontology: Series A,* 57, no. 7 (2002): M428–M432. doi.org/10.1093/gerona/57.7.M428.

Barba, B. E. (1995). "The Positive Influence of Animals: Animal-Assisted Therapy." *Acute Care Clinical Nurse Specialist* 9, no. 4 (1995): 199–202. doi:10.1097/00002800-199507000-00005.

Bardill, Norine, and Sally Hutchinson. "Animal-Assisted Therapy with Hospitalized Adolescents." *Journal of Child and Adolescent Psychiatric Nursing* 10, no. 1 (January 1997): 17–24. doi:10.1111/j.1744-6171.1997.tb00208.x.

Barker, S. B., J. S. Knisely, C. M. Schubert, J. D. Green, and S. Ameringer. "The Effect of an Animal-Assisted Intervention on Anxiety and Pain in Hospitalized Children." *Anthrozoos* 28, no. 1 (2015): 101–112.

Barker, Sandra B., and Aaron R. Wolen. "The Benefits of Human-Companion Animal Interaction: A Review." *Journal of Veterinary Medical Education* 35, no. 4 (2008): 487–95. doi:10.3138/jvme.35.4.487.

Barker, Sandra B., and Kathryn S. Dawson. "The Effects of Animal-Assisted Therapy on Anxiety Ratings of Hospitalized Psychiatric Patients." *Psychiatric Services* 49, no. 6 (1998): 797–801. doi:10.1176/ps.49.6.797.

Barker, Sandra B., and Randolph T. Barker. "The Human-Canine Bond: Closer than Family Ties?" *Journal of Mental Health Counseling* 10, no. 1 (1988): 46–56.

Barker, Sandra B., Randolph T. Barker, Nancy L. McCain, and Christine M. Schubert. "A Randomized Crossover Exploratory Study of the Effect of Visiting Therapy Dogs on College Student Stress Before Final Exams." *Anthrozoös* 29, no. 1 (2016): 35–46. doi:10.1080/08927936.2015.1069988.

Barker, Sandra B., Christopher S. Rogers, John W. Turner, Ariane S. Karpf, and H. Marie Suthers-McCabe. "Benefits of Interacting with Companion Animals: A Bibliography of Articles Published in Refereed Journals During the Past 5 Years." *American Behavioral Scientist* 47, no. 1 (September 2003), 94–99. doi: 10.1177/0002764203255215

Barker, Sandra B., Janet S. Knisely, Nancy L. McCain, and Al M. Best. "Measuring Stress and Immune Response in Healthcare Professionals Following Interaction with a Therapy Dog: A Pilot Study." *Psychological Reports* 96, no. 3 (2005): 713–29. doi:10.2466/pr0.96.3.713-729.

Barker, Sandra B., Janet S. Knisely, Nancy L. McCain, Christine M. Schubert, and Anand K. Pandurangi. "Exploratory Study of Stress-Buffering Response Patterns from Interac-tion with a Therapy Dog." *Anthrozoös* 23, no. 1 (2010): 79–91. doi:10.2752/175303710x12627079939341.

Barker, Sandra B., Randolph T. Barker, and Christine M. Schubert. "Therapy Dogs on Campus: A Counseling Outreach Activity for Students Preparing for Final Exams." *Journal of College Counseling* 20 (2017): 278–88. doi:10.1002/jocc.12075.

Bausum, Ann. *Sergeant Stubby: How a Stray Dog and His Best Friend Helped Win World War I and Stole the Heart of a Nation.* Washington, D.C.: National Geographic, 2014.

Baynes, Ernest. "Our Animal Allies in the World War." *Harpers Monthly,* January 1921: 70.

Beck, A. M., and A. H. Katcher. "Future Directions in Human-Animal Bond Research." *The American Behavioral Scientist,* vol. 47, no. 1 (2003): 79–93. http://journals.sagepub.com/doi/abs/10.1177/0002764203255214

Beck, A. M., and A. H. Katcher. "A New Look at Pet-Facilitated Therapy." *Journal of the American Veterinary Medical Association* 184, no. 4 (February 15, 1984), 414–21.

Beck, Jim. "The Five Secrets of Storytelling for Social Change." *Forbes,* August 1, 2013. https://www.forbes.com/sites/skollworldforum/2013/08/01/the-5-secrets-of-storytelling-for-social-change/2/#65d17b77532a.

Beetz, Andrea, Kerstin Uvnäs-Moberg, Henri Julius, and Kurt Kotrschal. "Psychosocial and Psychophysiological Effects of Human-Animal Interactions: The Possible Role of Oxytocin." *Frontiers in Psychology* 3 (2012): 234. doi:10.3389/fpsyg.2012.00234.

Bekoff, Marc. *The Emotional Lives of Animals: A Leading Scientist Explores Animal Joy, Sorrow, and Empathy—And Why They Matter.* Novato, CA: New World Library, 2008.

Berwick, Donald M. "Disseminating Innovations in Health Care." *JAMA* 289, no. 15 (2003): 1969–1975. doi:10.1001/jama.289.15.1969.

Binfet, John-Tyler. "The Effects of Group-Administered Canine Therapy on University Students' Wellbeing: A Randomized Controlled Trial." *Anthrozoös* 30, no. 3 (2017): 397–414.

Blazina, Christopher, Guler Boyraz, and David Shen-Miller, eds. *The Psychology of the Human-Animal Bond: A Resource for Clinicians and Researchers.* New York: Springer, 2011.

Blum, Nava, and Elizabeth Fee. "Howard A. Rusk (1901–1989): From Military Medicine to Comprehensive Rehabilitation." *American Journal of Public Health* 98 (2008): 256–57.

Bonaparte, Marie. *Topsy: The Story of a Golden-Haired Chow.* New Brunswick, NJ: Transaction Publishers, 1994.

Boni, Sarah Elizabeth. "Anthropomorphism: How It Affects the Human-Canine Bond." *Journal of Applied Companion Animal Behavior* 2 (2008): 16–21. http://www.associationofanimalbehaviorprofessionals.com/vol2no1.pdf.

Borrego, Javier L., Luis R. Franco, Maria A. Perea Mediavilla, Nuria Blanco Pinero, Arcadui Tejada Roldan, and Alfonso Blanco Picabia. (2014). "Animal-Assisted Interventions: Review of Current Status and Future Challenges." *International Journal of Psychology and Psychological Therapy* 14, no. 1 (2014): 85–101. http://www.ijpsy.com/volume n14/num1/376/animal-assisted-interventions-review-of-EN.pdf.

Bostridge, Mark. *Florence Nightingale: The Making of an Icon.* New York: Farrar, Straus and Giroux, 2008.

Bowlby, J. *Attachment and Loss: Attachment* (Vol. 1). New York: Basic Books, 1969.

Bowlby, J. "Attachment and Loss: Retrospect and Prospect." *American Journal of Orthopsychiatry* 52, no. 4 (1982): 664–78.

Bragg, J. Jeffrey. "Leonhard Seppala, All-Time Great of Alaskan Dog Drivers," 2003, updated 2005. http://www.seppalakennels.com/articles/leonhardseppala.htm.

Braitman, Laurel. "Dog Complex: Analyzing Freud's Relationship with His Pets." October 23, 2014. https://www.fastcompany.com/3037493/dog-complex-analyzing-freuds-relationship-with-his-pets Fast Company.

Brambell, Roger. *Report of the Technical Committee to Enquire into the Welfare of Animals Kept Under Intensive Livestock Husbandry Systems.* London: H. M. Stationery Office, 1965. http://edepot.wur.nl/134379.

Braun, Carie, Teresa Stangler, Jennifer Narveson, and Sandra Pettingell. "Animal-Assisted Therapy as a Pain Relief Intervention for Children." *Complementary Therapies in Clinical Practice* 15, no. 2 (2009): 105–09. doi:10.1016/j.ctcp.2009.02.008.

Bray, Emily E., Mary D. Sammel, Dorothy L. Cheney, James A. Serpell, and Robert M. Seyfarth. "Effects of Maternal Investment, Temperament, and Cognition on Guide Dog Success." *Proceedings of the National Academy of Sciences* 114 (2017): 9128–33. doi:10.1073/pnas.1704303114.

Brickel, Clark M. "Pet-Facilitated Psychotherapy: A Theoretical Explanation via Attention Shifts." *Psychological Reports* 50 (1982): 71–74. http://journals.sagepub.com/doi/10.2466/pr0.1982.50.1.71.

Brodie, Sarah J., Francis C. Biley, and Michael Shewring. "An Exploration of the Potential Risks Associated with Using Pet Therapy in Healthcare Settings." *Journal of Clinical Nursing* 11, no. 4 (2002): 444–56. doi:10.1046/j.1365-2702.2002.00628.x.

Browe, Amanda. *From the Archives: Red Cross Dogs.* American Red Cross, April 21, 2014. https://redcrosschat.org/2014/04/21/from-the-archives-red-cross-dogs/.

Brusher, E. A. "Combat and Operational Stress Control." *International Journal of Emergency Mental Health* 9, no. 2 (2007): 111–22. https://www.omicsonline.org/open-access/new-crisis-and-stress-management-programme-launched.pdf.

Burke, Shanna L., and Dorothea Iannuzzi. "Animal-Assisted Therapy for Children and Adolescents with Autism Spectrum Disorders." In *Animals in Social Work,* edited by T. Ryan. London: Palgrave Macmillan. https://doi.org/10.1057/9781137372291_8.

Bustad, L. K. "How Animals Make People Human and Humane." *Modern Veterinary Practice* 60 (1979): 707–10.

Bustad, L. K. "Reflections on the Human-Animal Bond." *Journal of the American Veterinary Medical Association* 208, no. 2 (1996): 203–5.

Byrne, Peter. "Freud's Dogs." June 4, 2012. http://www.swans.com/library/art18/pbyrne183.html.

Calcaterra, Valeria, Pierangelo Veggiotti, Clara Palestrini, Valentina De Giorgis, Roberto Raschetti, Massimiliano Tumminelli, Simonetta Mencherini, Francesca Papotti, Catherine Klersy, Riccardo Albertini, Selene Ostuni, and Gloria Pelizzo. "Post-Operative Benefits of Animal-Assisted Therapy in Pediatric Surgery: A Randomised Study." *PLoS One* 10, no 6 (June 3, 2015):e0125813. doi:10.1371/journal.pone.0125813.

Calvo, P., J. R. Fortuny, S. Guzmán, C. Macías, J. Bowen, M. L. García, O. Orejas, F. Molins, A. Tvarijonaviciute, J. J. Cerón, A. Bulbena, and J. Fatjó. "Animal Assisted Therapy (AAT) Program as a Useful Adjunct to Conventional Psychosocial Rehabilitation for Patients with Schizophrenia: Results of a Small-scale Randomized Controlled Trial." *Frontiers in Psychology* 7 (2016): 631. doi: 10.3389/fpsyg.2016.00631.

Campbell, Joseph. *The Hero with a Thousand Faces.* Princeton, NJ: Princeton University Press, 1949.

Caprilli, Simona, and Andrea Messeri. "Animal-Assisted Activity at A. Meyer Children's Hospital: A Pilot Study." *Evidence-Based Complementary and Alternative Medicine* 3, no. 3 (2006): 379–83. doi:10.1093/ecam/nel029.

Centers for Disease Control and Prevention. "About Diphtheria." Last updated January 15, 2016. https://www.cdc.gov/diphtheria/about/index.html.

Centers for Disease Control and Prevention. "Diphtheria." In. Updated November 9, 2015. CDC.gov/vaccines/pubs/pinkbook/dip/html.

Centers for Disease Control and Prevention. "Hospital Utilization (in Non-Federal Short-Stay Hospitals)." Updated May 3, 2017. http://www.cdc.gov/nchs/fastats/hospital.htm.

Centers for Disease Control and Prevention. "Iditarod: Celebrating the 'Great Race of Mercy' to Stop Diphtheria Outbreak in Alaska." Updated January 3, 2018. https://www.cdc.gov/about/24-7/savinglives/diphtheria/index.html

Centers for Disease Control and Prevention. "Immunization: The Basics." Updated March 10, 2017. https://www.cdc.gov/vaccines/vac-gen/imz-basics.htm

Centers for Disease Control and Prevention. "Indicators." Accessed May 4, 2018. https://www.cdc.gov/eval/indicators/index.htm

Centers for Disease Control and Prevention. "Keeping You Safe 24-7." Updated December 5, 2017. https:// www.cdc.gov/about/24-7/savinglives.

Centers for Disease Control and Prevention. "One Health Basics." Updated April 3, 2018. https://www.cdc.gov/onehealth/basics/index.html.

Centers for Disease Control and Prevention. "One Health Initiative." Accessed May 4, 2018. http://www.onehealthinitiative.com/mission.php.

Chandler, Cynthia. "Animal-Assisted Therapy in Counseling and School Settings." *ERIC/CASS Digest,* October 2010, 1–8. https://files.eric.ed.gov/fulltext/ED459404.pdf.

Chandler, Cynthia, Torey Portrie-Bethke, Casey Minton, Delini Fernando, and Dana O'Callaghan. "Matching Animal-Assisted Therapy Techniques and Intentions with Counseling Guiding Theories." *Journal of Mental Health Counseling* 32, no. 4 (2010): 354–74.

Chandler, Cynthia K. *Animal-Assisted Therapy in Counseling,* 2nd ed. New York: Routledge, 2012.

Children's Health. "Facility Dogs." Accessed April 30, 2018. https://www.childrens.com/patient-families/resources-for-your-child/child-life/pet-assisted-therapy/meet-the-dogs/facility-dogs.

Chow Chow Club. "A Chow Chow's Personality and Habits." Accessed September 13, 2017. https://chowclub.org/ccci/content/view/23/35/.

Chowtales. "Why Did Chows Change." Accessed May 15, 2018. https://chowtales.com/page-two/.

Chubak, Jessica, and Rene Hawkes. "Animal-Assisted Activities." *Journal of Pediatric Oncology Nursing* 33, no. 4 (2016): 289–96.

Chumley, P. R. "Historical Perspectives of the Human-Animal Bond Within the Department of Defense." *U.S. Army Medical Department Journal* 2 (2012): 18–20.

Chur-Hansen, A., M. McArthur, H. Winefield, E. Hanieh, and S. Hazel. "Animal-Assisted Interventions in Children's Hospitals: A Critical Review of the Literature." *Anthrozoös* 27 no. 1 (2014): 5–18. doi: 10.2752/175303714X13837396326251.

Chur-Hansen, Anna, Cindy Stern, and Helen Winefield. "Gaps in the Evidence About Companion Animals and Human Health: Some Suggestions for Progress." *International Journal of Evidence-Based Healthcare* 8 no. 3 (2010): 140–46.

Clark, Blake, and Morris Frank. *First Lady of The Seeing Eye.* New York: Henry Holt, 1957.

Cleveland Museum of Natural History. *Balto and the Legacy of the Serum Run* [brochure]. Cleveland: Author, not dated. https://www.cmnh.org/CMNH/media/CMNH_Media/Balto/Balto-and-the-Legacy-of-the-Serum-Run.pdf

Cole, K., A. Gawlinski, N. Steers, and J. Kotlerman. "Animal Assisted Therapy in Patients Hospitalized with Heart Failure." *American Journal of Critical Care* 16 no. 6 (2007): 575–85.

Cole, Kathie M., and Anna Gawlinski. "Animal-Assisted Therapy in the Intensive Care Unit." *Nursing Clinics of North America* 30, no. 3 (September 1995): 529–37.

Coley, Herbert A. "Overarching Guidance on the Use of Animals in the Healthcare Setting (Service Animals, Animal Assisted Therapies, and Animal Assisted Activities)," Memorandum, U.S. Army, January 30, 2012. https://www.army.mil/e2/c/downloads/250935.pdf.

Cook, Edward Tyas. *The Life of Florence Nightingale,* Vols. 1 and 2. New York: Macmillan, 1913.

Coppock, Mike. "The Race to Save Nome." *American History* 41, no. 3 (2006): 56–63.

Coren, Stanley. "Florence Nightingale: The Dog and the Dream." *Canine Corner Blog, Psychology Today,* June 15, 2010. https://www.psychologytoday.com/blog/canine-corner/201006/florence-nightingale-the-dog-and-the-dream.

Coren, Stanley. "Foreword." In *Handbook on Animal-Assisted Therapy,* 4th ed., edited by Aubrey H. Fine, xix–xxii. Amsterdam: Elsevier/Academic Press, 2015.

Coren, Stanley. "How Therapy Dogs Almost Never Came to Exist." *Canine Corner Blog, Psychology Today,* February 11, 2013. https://

www.psychologytoday.com/blog/canine-corner/201302/how-therapy-dogs-almost-never-came-exist.

Coren, Stanley. *Pawprints of History*. New York: Free Press, 2002.

Correa, Julio E. "The Dog's Sense of Smell." Alabama Cooperative Extension System, February 2016. https://www.aces.edu/pubs/docs/U/UNP-0066/UNP-0066.pdf.

Corrigan, P. W., B. G. Druss, and D. A. Perlick. "The Impact of Mental Illness Stigma on Seeking and Participating in Mental Health Care." *Psychological Science in the Public Interest* 15 no. 2 (2014): 37–70.

Corson, S. A., E. O. Corson, P. H. Gwynne, and L. E. Arnold. "Pet-Facilitated Psychotherapy in a Hospital Setting." *Current Psychiatric Therapies* 15 (1975): 277–86.

Corson, S. A., L. E. Arnold, P. H. Gwynne, and E. O. L. Corson. "Pet Dogs as Nonverbal Communication Links in Hospital Psychiatry." *Comprehensive Psychiatry* 18 (1977): 61–72.

Cox, Mark. "Dogs of War: The First Aiders on Four Legs." November 10, 2014. http://blogs.redcross.org.uk/first-aid/2014/11/dogs-war-first-aiders-four-legs/.

Craigon, Peter J., Pru Hobson-West, Gary C. W. England, Chantelle Whelan, Emma Lethbridge, and Lucy Asher. "'She's a Dog at the End of the Day': Guide Dog Owners' Perspectives on the Behaviour of Their Guide Dog." *PLoS One* 12, no. 4 (2017, April 19). https://doi.org/10.1371/journal.pone.0176018.

Creagan, Edward T., Brent A. Bauer, Barbara S. Thomley, and Jessica M. Borg. "Animal-Assisted Therapy at Mayo Clinic: The Time Is Now." *Complementary Therapies in Clinical Practice* 21, no. 2 (2015): 101–04. doi:10.1016/j.ctcp.2015.03.002.

Crossman, Molly. "Effects of Interactions with Animals on Human Psychological Distress." *Journal of Clinical Psychology* 73, no. 7 (2017): 761–84.

Cukor, Judith, Josh Spitalnick, JoAnn Difede, Albert Rizzo, and Barbara O. Rothbaum. "Emerging Treatments for PTSD." *Clinical Psychology Review* 29 (2009): 715–26. doi:10.1016/j.cpr.2009.09.001.

Cunningham, David. "Top Dogs: September is National Service Dog Month." Defense Visual Information Distribution Service. Accessed September 21, 2019. https://www.dvidshub.net.news/262500/top-dogs-september-national-service-dog-month

Dalton, Clive. "Farm Dogs." In *Te Ara—The Encyclopedia of New Zealand*, November 24, 2008. https://teara.govt.nz/mi/farm-dogs/print

D'Amore, Arcangelo R. T. "Introduction." In *William Alanson White: The Washington Years 1903–1937. The Contributions to Psychiatry, Psychoanalysis and Mental Health by Dr. White While Superintendent of Saint Elizabeths Hospital*, 1–12. Washington, D.C.: National Institute of Mental Health, 1976.

Delta Society. *Standards of Practice for Animal-Assisted Activities and Animal-Assisted Therapy*. Renton, WA: Delta Society, 1996.

Delta Society. *Student Manual 2008*. Renton, WA: Delta Society, 2008.

Department of Defense. "Demographics: Profile of the Military Community," 2012. http://www.militaryonesource.mil/12038/MOS/Reports/2012_Demographics_Report.pdf.

Department of Defense. *Human-Animal Bond: Principles and Guidelines*. Washington, D.C.: Author, 2003. http://www17.us.archive.org/stream/ost-military-medical-tbmed4/tbmed4_djvu.txt.

Department of Health and Human Services. *Mental Health: A Report of the Surgeon General*. Rockville, MD: Center for Mental Health Services, National Institutes of Health, 1999.

Department of Justice. "Service Animals," 2011. http://www.ada.gov/service_animals_2010.htm.

Dickens, Charles. *American Notes*. London: Chapman Hall Ltd., 1913. https://www.gutenberg.org/files/675/675-h/675-h.htm.

Dingfelder, Sadie F. "The Military's War on Stigma." *Monitor* 40, no. 6 (2009): 52. http://www.apa.org/monitor/2009/06/stigma-war.aspx.

"'Dirty Old London': A History of the Victorians' Infamous Filth." NPR author interview, March 12, 2015. http://www.npr.org/2015/03/12/392332431/dirty-old-london-a-history-of-the-victorians-infamous-filth.

Disalvo, Heidi, Donna Haiduven, Nancy Johnson, Valentine V. Reyes, Carmen P. Hench, Rosemary Shaw, and David A. Stevens. "Who Let the Dogs Out? Infection Control Did: Utility of Dogs in Health Care Settings and Infection Control Aspects." *American Journal of Infection Control* 34, no. 5 (June 2006): 301–07. doi:10.1016/j.ajic.2005.06.005.

Doolittle, Hilda. *Tribute to Freud*. New York: New Directions Books, 1974.

Dossey, Barbara. "Florence Nightingale: Mystic, Visionary, Healer." Lecture Transcript, Washington National Cathedral, August 12, 2001. http://www.dosseydossey.com/barbara/floranceLecture.html.

Dossey, Barbara. *Florence Nightingale: Mystic, Visionary, Reformer*. Philadelphia: F. A. Davis, 2009.

Dossey, Barbara Montgomery, Louise C. Selanders, Deva-Marie Beck, and Alex Attewell. *Florence Nightingale Today: Healing,*

Leadership, Global Action. Silver Spring, MD: American Nurses Association, 2005.

Draper, R. J., G. J. Gerber, and E. M. Layng. "Defining the Role of Pet Animals in Psychotherapy." *Psychiatric Journal of the University of Ottawa* 15 (1990): 169–72.

Duncan, Susan L. "APIC State-of-the-Art Report: The Implications of Service Animals in Health Care Settings." *American Journal of Infection Control* 28 (2000): 170–80. http://dx.doi.org/10.1016/S0196-6553(00)90025-7.

Dunham, Mike. "Emily's Mission: Dispensing the Famous Serum." *Alaska Dispatch News,* March 14, 2011; updated September 29, 2016. https://www.adn.com/iditarod/article/emilys-mission-dispensing-famous-nome-serum/2011/03/15/.

Dyer, Walter A. "Wanted: More Red Cross Dogs for America." *The Red Cross Magazine* 12, no. 10 (November 1917).

Edmundson, Mark. *The Death of Sigmund Freud: The Legacy of His Last Days.* New York: Bloomsbury, 2007.

Elbogen, E. B., H. R. Wagner, S. C. Johnson, P. Kinneer, H. Kang, J. J. Vasterling, et al. "Are Iraq and Afghanistan Veterans Using Mental Health Services? New Data from a National Random-Sample Survey." *Psychiatric Services* 64, no. 2 (2013): 134–41.

Ellis, Harold. "Edwin Klebs: Discoverer of the Bacillus of Diphtheria." *British Journal of Hospital Medicine* 74, no. 11 (2005): 641.

Ensminger, John. "Red Cross, Iron Cross: Ambulance Dogs in World War I." July 16, 2011. http://doglawreporter.blogspot.com/2011/07/red-cross-iron-cross-ambulance-dogs-in.html.

Ensminger, John J. *Service and Therapy Dogs in American Society: Science, Law and the Evolution of Canine Caregivers.* Springfield, IL: Charles C. Thomas, 2010.

Esteres, S. W., and T. Stakes. "Social Effects of a Dog's Presence on Children with Disabilities." *Anthrozoos* 21, no. 1 (2008): 5–15.

Eustis, Dorothy Harrison. "The Seeing Eye." *The Saturday Evening Post,* November 15, 1927.

Feldman, Steven. "The Power of the Pet Effect." Presented at the Pet Partners Professionalizing the Passion Conference, September 2017. https://petpartners.org/wp-content/uploads/2017/01/Steve-Feldman_conf2017.pdf.

Fick, K. M. "The Influence of an Animal on Social Interactions of Nursing Home Residents in a Group Setting." *American Journal of Occupational Therapy* 47, no. 6 (1993): 529–34. doi:10.5014/ajot.47.6.529.

Fike, Laurie, Cecilia Najera, and David Dougherty. "Occupational Therapists as Dog Handlers: The Collective Experience with Animal-Assisted Therapy in Iraq." *U.S. Army Medical Department Journal* (2012, Apr-Jun): 51–54.

Fine, Aubrey, Philip Tedeshi, and Erica Elvove. "Forward Thinking: The Evolving Field of Human-Animal Interactions." In *Handbook on Animal-Assisted Therapy,* 4th ed., edited by Aubrey H. Fine, 21–35. Amsterdam: Elsevier/Academic Press, 2015.

Fine, Aubrey H. "Incorporating Animal-Assisted Interventions into Psychotherapy." In *Handbook on Animal-Assisted Therapy,* 4th ed., edited by Aubrey H. Fine, 141–55. Amsterdam: Elsevier/Academic Press, 2015.

Fine, Aubrey H. "Standing the Test of Time: Reflecting on the Relevance Today of Levinson's Pet-Oriented Child Psychotherapy." *Clinical Child Psychology and Psychiatry* 22 no. 1 (2017): 9–15.

Fine, Aubrey H., and Alan M. Beck. "Understanding Our Kinship with Animals: Input for Health Care Professionals Interested in the Human-Animal Bond." In *Handbook on Animal-Assisted Therapy,* 4th ed., edited by Aubrey H. Fine, 3–10. Amsterdam, Elsevier Academic Press, 2015.

Fine, Aubrey H. (Ed.). *Handbook on Animal-Assisted Therapy: Foundations and Guidelines for Animal-Assisted Interventions* (4th ed.). San Diego, CA: Elsevier, Inc., 2015.

Fine, Aubrey H. (Ed.). *Handbook on Animal-Assisted Therapy: Theoretical Foundations and Guidelines for Practice* (3rd ed.). New York: Elsevier, 2010.

Francis, Gloria, Jean T. Turner, and Suzanne B. Johnson. "Domestic Animal Visitation as Therapy with Adult Home Residents." *International Journal of Nursing Studies* 22, no. 3 (1985): 201–06. doi:10.1016/0020-7489(85)90003-3.

Frank, Morris S. Letter to Miss Dorothy Harrison Eustis, November 9, 1927. http://www.seeingeye.org/assets/pdfs/history/Frankfranks-letter.pdf.

Frankel, Rebecca. "The Dog Whisperer: How a British Colonel Altered the Battlefields of World War I, and Why His Crusade Still Resonates Today." *Foreign Policy* 208 (Sep/Oct 2014): 90–3, 95, 98. http://foreignpolicy.com/2014/10/22/the-dog-whisperer/

Frankel, Rebecca. "Dogs at War: Smoky, A Healing Presence for Wounded WWII Soldiers." *National Geographic,* May 27, 2014. Accessed June 30, 2018. https://news.nationalgeographic.com/news/2014/05/140520-dogs-war-canines-soldiers-military-healing-yorkshire-terrier-smoky/

Frankel, Rebecca. *War Dogs: Tales of Heroism, History and Love.* New York: St. Martin's Press, 2016.

Freud, Anna. "Foreword." In *Topsy: The Story of*

a Golden-Haired Chow, by Marie Bonaparte, pp. 358–362. New Brunswick, NJ: Transaction Publishers, 1994.

Freud, Anna. Letter to Sigmund Freud, July 7, 1921.

Freud, Martin. *Glory Reflected: Sigmund Freud— Man and Father.* Melbourne, Australia: Angus and Robertson, 1957.

Freud, Sigmund. *Introduction to Psychoanalysis,* 1917 electronic version. http://www.gutenberg.org/ebooks/38219.

Freud Museum London. "Glossary of Terms." Accessed August 3, 2017. https://www.freud.org.uk/education/topic/10575/subtopic/74476/.

Friedman, Susan Stanford, ed. *Analyzing Freud: The Letters of H. D. Bryher and Their Circle.* New York: New Direction Books, 2002.

Friedmann, Erika, and Heesook Son. "The Human-Companion Animal Bond: How Humans Benefit." *Veterinary Clinics of North America: Small Animal Practice* 39, no. 2 (2009): 293–326. doi:10.1016/j.cvsm.2008.10.015.

Friedmann, Erika, Heesook Son, and Chia-Chun Tsai. "The Animal/Human Bond." In *Handbook on Animal-Assisted Therapy,* 3rd ed., edited by Aubrey H. Fine, 85–107. Amsterdam, Elsevier Academic Press, 2010.

Friedmann, Erika, Sue A. Thomas, Linda K. Cook, Chia-Chun Tsai, and Sandra J. Picot. "A Friendly Dog as Potential Moderator of Cardiovascular Response to Speech in Older Hypertensives." *Anthrozoös* 20, no. 1 (2007): 51–63. doi:10.2752/089279307780216605.

"Funeral of Miss Nightingale." *The Morning Post,* August 22, 1910. As quoted in *The Life and Times of Florence Nightingale Blog.* Accessed April 28, 2018. https://lifeandtimesofflorencenightingale.wordpress.com/newspaper-and-magazine-articles/the-morning-post-august-22-1910/.

Gagnon, Johanne, France Bouchard, Marie Landry, Marthe Belles-Isles, Martine Fortier, and Lise Fillion. "Implementing a Hospital-Based Animal Therapy Program for Children with Cancer: A Descriptive Study." *Canadian Oncology Nursing Journal* 14, no. 4 (2004): 217–22. doi:10.5737/1181912x144217222.

Gammonley, Judy, Ann R. Howie, Sherry Kirwin, Susan A. Zapf, Jeanne Frye, Gertrude Freeman, and Robbye Stuart-Russell. *Animal-Assisted Therapy: Therapeutic Interventions.* Renton, WA: Delta Society, 1997.

Gay, Peter. *Freud: A Life for Our Time.* New York: Norton, 1988.

Genosko, Gary. "Introduction." In *Topsy: The Story of a Golden-Haired Chow,* by Marie Bonaparte. New Brunswick, NJ: Transaction Publishers, 1994.

Germain, Sarah M., Karlene D. Wilkie, Virginia M. K. Milbourne, and Jennifer Theule. "Animal-Assisted Psychotherapy and Trauma: A Meta-Analysis." *Anthrozoös* 31, no. 2 (2018): 141–164.

"German Shepherd Dogs." *Scientific American* 71, no. 15 (October 13, 1894): 232. http://www.jstor.org/stable/26114738.

Gifford, J. T. *Constance and Cap, the Shepherd's Dog: A Remembrance.* Harrison, 1861.

Gill, Gillian. *Nightingales: The Extraordinary Upbringing and Curious Life of Miss Florence Nightingale.* New York: Random House, 2004.

Gilmer, Mary Jo, Marissa N. Baudino, Anna Tielsch Goddard, Donna C. Vickers, Terrah Foster Akard. "Animal-Assisted Therapy in Pediatric Palliative Care." *Nursing Clinics of North America* 51, no. 3 (2016): 381–95.

Ginex, Pamela, Mary Montefusco, Glenn Zecco, Nicole Trocchia Mattessich, Jacquelyn Burns, Jane Hedal-Siegel, Jane Kopelman, and Kay See Tan. "Animal-Facilitated Therapy Program: Outcomes from Caring Canines, a Program for Patients and Staff on an Inpatient Surgical Oncology Unit." *Clinical Journal of Oncology Nursing* 22, no. 2 (2018): 193–98.

Giuliano, K. K., E. Bloniasz, and J. Bell. "Implementation of a Pet Visitation Program in Critical Care." *Critical Care Nurse* 19, no. 3 (1999): 43–50.

Glenk, Lisa. "Current Perspectives on Therapy Dog Welfare in Animal-Assisted Interventions." *Animals* 7, no. 2 (2017): 7. doi:10.3390/ani7020007.

Gloria Dei Garland. "Creature Care." Accessed June 18, 2018. http://gloriadeigarland.com/about-us/creature-care/.

Glucksman, Myron L. "The Dog's Role in the Analyst's Consulting Room." *Journal of the American Academy of Psychoanalysis and Dynamic Psychiatry* 33, no. 4 (2005): 611–18.

Goddard, Anna Tielsch, and Mary Jo Gilmer. "The Role and Impact of Animals with Pediatric Patients." *Pediatric Nursing* 41, no. 2 (March-April 2015): 65–69. https://www.pediatricnursing.net/ce/2017/article4102 6571.pdf.

Graham, Effie, Jackie Pflaum, and Elfirda Nord. *With a Dauntless Spirit: Alaska Nursing in Dog-Team Days.* Fairbanks: University of Alaska Press, 2003.

Grandin, Temple, and Catherine Johnson. *Animals in Translation: Using the Mysteries of Autism to Decode Animal Behavior.* Orlando, FL: Harvest, 2005.

Grandin, Temple, and Catherine Johnson. *Animals Make Us Human: Creating the Best Life for Animals.* Boston: Mariner Books, 2010.

Granger, Ben P., and Lori R. Kogan. "Characteristics of Animal-Assisted Therapy/Activity in Specialized Settings." In *Handbook on Animal-Assisted Therapy: Theoretical Foundations and Guidelines for Practice*, edited by Aubrey Fine, 263–85. New York: Academic Press, 2006.

Granger, Ben P., Lori Kogan, Jennifer Fitchett, and Kim Helmer. "A Human-Animal Intervention Team Approach to Animal-Assisted Therapy." *Anthrozoös* 11, no. 3 (1998): 172–76. doi:10.2752/089279398787000689.

Green, Susie. "Freud's Dream Companions." *The Guardian*, March 22, 2002. https://www.theguardian.com/theguardian/2002/mar/23/weekend7.weekend3.

Greg, W. R. *Why Are Women Redundant?* London: N. Trubner & Co., 1869.

Gregg, Brian T. "Crossing the Berm: An Occupational Therapist's Perspective on Animal-Assisted Therapy in a Deployed Environment." *U.S. Army Medical Department Journal* 2 (April-June 2012): 55–56.

Griffin, James A., Sandra McCune, Valerie Maholmes, and Karyl J. Hurley. "Scientific Research on Human-Animal Interaction: A Framework for Future Studies." In *Animals in Our Lives: Human-Animal Interaction in Family, Community and Therapeutic Settings*, edited by Peggy McCardle, Sandra McCune, James A. Griffin, Layla Esposito, and Lisa S. Freund, 11–22. Baltimore, MD: Paul H. Brookes Publishing Co., 2011.

Grinker, Roy, Sr. "A Memoir of My Psychoanalytic Education." *Psychoanalytic Education* 4 (1985), 3–12.

Grinker, Roy R., Jr. "My Father's Analysis with Sigmund Freud." *Annual of Psychoanalysis* 29 (2001): 35–47.

Grinker, Roy R., Sr. "Reminiscences of a Personal Contact with Freud." *American Journal of Orthopsychiatry* 10 (1940): 850–854.

Gustkey, Earl. "The Iditarod: Mushers Follow Call of the Wild, but Their Dogs' 1,000-Mile Race Across Alaska's Frozen Wastes Is Enough to Give Anyone Paws," *Los Angeles Times*, March 24, 1986. http://articles.latimes.com/1986-03-24/sports/sp-126_1_lead-dog

H. D. and Bryher Papers, Special Collection Department, Bryn Mawr College Library. Accessed May 4, 2018.

HABRI Central. Home page. Accessed June 19, 2018. https://habricentral.org/.

Haidich, A. B. "Meta-Analysis in Medical Research." *Hippokratia* 14, suppl. 1 (2010), 29–37.

Haladay, J. "Animal Assisted Therapy for PWA's: Bringing a Sense of Connection." *AIDS Patient Care* 3, no. 1 (1989): 38–9.

Halcomb, Ralph, and Mary Meacham. "Effectiveness of an Animal-Assisted Therapy Program in an In-patient Psychiatric Program." *Anthrozoos* 2, no. 4 (1989): 259–64.

Hansen, Kristine M., Cathy J. Messinger, Mara M. Baun, and Mary Megel. "Companion Animals Alleviating Distress in Children." *Anthrozoös* 12, no. 3 (1999): 142–48. doi:10.2752/089279399787000264.

Harper, Carl M., Thomas S. Yan Dong, John Wright Thornhill, John Ready, Gregory W. Brick, and George Dyer. "Can Therapy Dogs Improve Pain and Satisfaction After Total Joint Arthroplasty? A Randomized Controlled Trial." *Clinical Orthopaedics and Related Research* 473, no. 1 (2014): 372–79. doi: 10.1007/s11999-014-3931-0.

Harris, Marilyn D., Joan M. Rinehart, and Jody Gerstman. "Animal-Assisted Therapy for the Homebound Elderly." *Holistic Nursing Practice* 8, no. 1 (1993): 27–37. doi:10.1097/0000 4650-199310000-00006.

Haughie, Elaine, Derek Milne, and Valerie Elliott. "An Evaluation of Companion Pets with Elderly Psychiatric Patients." *Behavioural Psychotherapy* 20, no. 4 (1992): 367–72. doi:10.1017/s0141347300017511.

Havey, Julia, Frances R. Vlasses, Peter H. Vlasses, Patti Ludwig-Beymer, and Diana Hackbarth. "The Effect of Animal-Assisted Therapy on Pain Medication Use After Joint Replacement." *Anthrozoös* 27, no. 3 (2014): 361–69. https://www.tandfonline.com/doi/abs/10.2752/175303714X13903827487962

Headquarters, Department of the Army. *Field Manual 4-02.51: Combat and Operational Stress Control.* Accessed November 15, 2017. https://fas.org/irp/doddir/army/fm4-02-51.pdf.

Hendrick, Ellwood. "Merciful Dogs of War." *The Red Cross Magazine* 12 (1917): 71–5.

Herzog, Harold. "The Research Challenge: Threats to the Validity of Animal-Assisted Therapy Studies and Suggestions for Improvement." In *Handbook on Animal-Assisted Therapy*, 4th ed., edited by Aubrey H. Fine, 408–13. San Diego: Academic Press, 2015.

Hoge, C. W., C. A. Castro, S. C. Messer, D. McGurk, D. I. Cotting, and R. L. Koffman. "Combat Duty in Iraq and Afghanistan, Mental Health Problems, and Barriers to Care." *New England Journal of Medicine* 351, no. 1 (2004): 13–22.

Holcomb, R., and M. Meacham. "Effectiveness of an Animal-Assisted Therapy Program in an Inpatient Psychiatric Unit." *Anthrozoos* 2, no. 4 (1989): 259–64.

Holland, Norman N. "H. D.'s Analysis with Freud." *PSYART Journal*, April 26, 2002. http://psyartjournal.com/article/show/n_holland-hds_analysis_with_freud.

Hooker, S. D., L. H. Freeman, and P. Stewart. "Pet Therapy Research: A Historical Review." *Holistic Nursing Practice* 16, no. 5 (2002):17-

23. https://www.researchgate.net/publication/11006382_Pet_therapy_research_A_historical_review.

Horowitz, Alexandra. *Inside of a Dog: What Dogs See, Smell, and Know.* New York: Scribner's, 2010.

Horowitz, Sala. "Animal-Assisted Therapy for Inpatients: Tapping the Unique Healing Power of the Human-Animal Bond." *Alternative and Complementary Therapies* 16, no. 6 (2010): 339–43. doi:10.1089/act.2010.16603.

Hosey, Geoff, and Vicky Melfi. "Human-Animal Interactions, Relationships and Bonds: A Review and Analysis of the Literature." *International Journal of Comparative Psychology* 27, no. 1 (2014). https://escholarship.org/uc/item/6955n8kd.

Houdek, Jennifer. "The Serum Run of 1925." *Lit Site Alaska.* Accessed October 7, 2017. http://www.litsite.org/index.cfm?section=Digital%20Archives&page=Land%20Sea%20Air&cat=Dog%20Mushing&contentid=2559&viewpost=2.

Howie, Ann. "Sample Goals and Methods." In *Standards of Practice for Animal-Assisted Activities and Animal-Assisted Therapy,* edited by Delta Society, 87–92. Renton, WA: Delta Society, 1996.

Howie, Ann R. *Teaming with Your Therapy Dog.* Lafayette, IN: Purdue University Press, 2015.

Human Animal Bond Research Institute. "Animal-Assisted Intervention for Post-Traumatic Stress Disorder (PTSD): A Systematic Review." Accessed June 15, 2018. https://habri.org/grants/projects/animal-assisted-intervention-for-post-traumatic-stress-disorder-ptsd-a-systematic-review.

Human Animal Bond Research Institute. "Family Physician Survey: Pets and Health." Accessed June 15, 2018. https://habri.org/2014-physician-survey.

Human Animal Bond Research Institute. "Healthy Aging: How the Human-Animal Bond Can Help." Accessed January 5, 2018. https://habri.org/research/healthy-aging.

Human Animal Bond Research Institute. "The Pet Effect." Accessed June 15, 2018. https://habri.org/the-pet-effect.

Human Animal Bond Research Institute. "Research: Understanding the Human-Animal Bond." Accessed June 15, 2018. https://habri.org/research/.

Humphrey, Elliott, and Lucien Warner. *Working Dogs: An Attempt to Produce a Strain of German Shepherd Which Combines Working Ability and Beauty of Conformation.* Baltimore: Johns Hopkins University Press, 1934. https://archive.org/details/workingdogsatte00elli

Hundley, J. "Pet Project: The Use of Pet Facilitated Therapy Among the Chronically Mentally Ill." *Journal of Psychosocial Nursing & Mental Health Services* 29, no. 6 (1991): 23–26.

Hunt, Melissa G., and Rachel R. Chizkov. "Are Therapy Dogs Like Xanax? Does Animal-Assisted Therapy Impact Processes Relevant to Cognitive Behavioral Psychotherapy?" *Anthrozoös* 27, no. 3 (2014): 457–69.

Hunt, Susan J., Lynette A. Hart, and Richard Gomulkiewicz. "Role of Small Animals in Social Interactions Between Strangers." *Journal of Social Psychology* 132 (1992): 245–56. doi:10.1080/00224545.1992.9922976.

Infection Control Today. "Transmission Prevention Cleaning Procedure Prevents Therapy Dogs Spreading MRSA to Children With Cancer." Accessed 10/29/2018, https://www.infectioncontroltoday.com/transmission-prevention/cleaning-procedure-prevents-therapy-dogs-spreading-mrsa-children-cancer

International Association of Human-Animal Interaction Organizations. *The IAHAIO Definitions for Animal Assisted interventions and Guidelines for Wellness of Animals Involved in AAI* [IAHAIO White Paper]. 2014; updated for 2018. http://iahaio.org/wp/wp-content/uploads/2018/04/iahaio_wp_updated-2018-final.pdf.

International Guide Dog Federation. "History of Guide Dogs," 2017. https://www.igdf.org.uk/about-us/facts-and-figures/history-of-guide-dogs/.

Jackson, Lee. *Dirty Old London: The Victorian Fight Against Filth.* New Haven, CT: Yale University Press, 2014.

Jager, Theodore F. *Scout, Red Cross and Army Dogs: A Historical Sketch of Dogs in the Great War and a Training Guide for the Rank and File of the United States Army.* Rochester, NY: Arrow Printing Company, 1917.

Jarolim, Edie. "Dogs and Psychoanalysis, Part 2: The Barking Cure." Willmydoghateme.com, January 24, 2012. http://willmydoghateme.com/pet-cetera/dogs-psychoanalysis-part-2-the-barking-cure.

Jenkins, M., A. Ruehrdanz, A. McCullough, K. Casillas, and J. D. Fluke. *Canines and Childhood Cancer: Examining the Effects of Therapy Dogs with Childhood Cancer Patients and Their Families.* Washington, D.C.: American Humane Association, 2012. https://www.americanhumane.org/app/uploads/2016/08/january2012clcompressed.pdf.

Johnson, Rebecca A., Johannes S. J. Odendaal, and Richard L. Meadows. "Animal-Assisted Interventions Research: Issues and Answers." *Western Journal of Nursing Research* 24, no. 4 (2002): 422–40. doi:10.1177/019459020240 04009.

The Joint Commission. "Revised Standard CTS. 01.01.01." In *Behavioral Health Care Accreditation Program.* Accessed January 5, 2018. https://www.jointcommission.org/assets/1/18/Post_BHC_CTS%20Chapter_20100630.pdf.

Jones, Edgar. "Shell Shocked." *Monitor on Psychology* 43, no. 6 (June 2012). http://www.apa.org/monitor/2012/06/shell-shocked.aspx.

Jones, Ernest. *The Life and Work of Sigmund Freud.* New York: Basic Books, 1975.

Jones, Kathleen. *Lunacy, Law, and Conscience, 1744–1845: The Social History of the Care of the Insane.* London: Routledge and Kegan Paul, 1955.

Kahn, Peter H. "Developmental Psychology and the Biophilia Hypothesis: Children's Affiliation with Nature." Developmental Review 17, no. 1 (1997): 1–61.

Kamioka, Hiroharu, Shinpei Okada, Kiichiro Tsutani, Hyuntae Park, Hiroyasu Okuizumi, Shuichi Handa, Takuya Oshio, Sang-Jun Park, Jun Kitayuguchi, Takafumi Abe, Takuya Honda, and Yoshiteru Mutohi. "Effectiveness of Animal-Assisted Therapy: A Systematic Review of Randomized Controlled Trials." *Complementary Therapies in Medicine* 22 (2014): 371–390. doi:10.1016/j.ctim.2013.12.016.

Kansas Historical Society. "Emily Morgan," 2013. https://www.kshs.org/kansapedia/emily-morgan/18267.

Kaplan, Melanie D. G. "Dogs Bring Relief to Soldiers: Operational Stress Control." *Bark* (March-May 2012): 53–55. http://melaniedgkaplan.com/MDGK_ARTICLES_files/Bark2.pdf.

Katcher, Aaron H., and E. Friedman. "Potential Health Value of Pet Ownership." *Compendium on Continuing Education for the Veterinarian* 2 (1980), 117–21.

Katcher, Aaron H., and M. Beck Alan. "Newer and Older Perspectives on the Therapeutic Effects of Animals and Nature." In *Handbook on Animal-Assisted Therapy,* 3rd ed., edited by Aubrey H. Fine, 49–58. Amsterdam, Elsevier Academic Press, 2010

Katz, Jon. *A Dog Year: Twelve Months, Four Dogs and Me.* New York: Random House, 2003.

Katz, Jon. *The New Work of Dogs: Tending to Life, Love, and Family.* New York: Random House, 2003.

Kazdin, A. E. "Establishing the Effectiveness of Animal-Assisted Therapies: Methodological Standards, Issues, and Strategies." In *How Animals Affect Us: Examining the Influence of Human-Animal Interactions on Child Development and Human Health,* edited by P. McCardle, S. McCune, J. A. Griffin, and V. Maholmes, pp. 35–51. Washington, D.C.: American Psychological Association.

Kehle, S. M., M. A. Polusny, M. Murdoch, C. R. Erbes, P. A. Arbisi, P. Thuras, P., and L. A. Meis. "Early Mental Health Treatment-Seeking Among U.S. National Guard Soldiers Deployed to Iraq." *Journal of Traumatic Stress* 23, no. 1 (2010): 33–40.

King, D. W., D. S. Vogt, and L. A. King. "Risk and Resilience Factors in the Etiology of Chronic PTSD." In *Early Interventions for Trauma and Traumatic Loss in Children and Adults: Evidence-Based Directions,* edited by B. T. Litz, 34–64. New York: Guilford Press, 2003.

King, L. J., L. R. Anderson, C. G. Blackmore, M. J. Blackwell, E. A. Lautner, L. C. Marcus, T. E. Meyer, T. P. Monath, J. E. Nave, J. Ohle, M. Pappaioanou, J. Sobota, W. S. Stokes, R. M. Davis, J. H. Glasser, R. K. Mahr. "Executive Summary of the AVMA One Health Initiative Task Force Report." *Journal of the American Veterinary Medical Association* 233, no. 2 (2009):259–61. doi:10.2460/javma.233.2.259.

Klein, Christopher. "Ten Things You May Not Know about Sigmund Freud." History.com, September 23, 2014. http://www.history.com/news/10-things-you-may-not-know-about-sigmund-freud.

Kleinman, Lawrence C. "To End an Epidemic: Lessons from the History of Diphtheria." *New England Journal of Medicine* 326 (1992): 773–77.

Knisely, Janet S., Sandra B. Barker, and Randolph T. Barker. "Research on Benefits of Canine-Assisted Therapy for Adults in Nonmilitary Settings." *US Army Medical Department Journal* (April-June 2012): 30–37. https://habricentral.org/resources/684/download/knisely_barker_barker-canine_assisted_therapy_in_nonmil_settings.pdf.

Knowles Bolton, Sarah. *Lives of Girls Who Became Famous.* Charleston, SC: BiblioLife, 2008 (originally published in 1914).

Kogan, Lori R., Ben P. Granger, Jennifer A. Fitchett, Kimberly A. Helmer, and Kaili J. Young. "The Human-Animal Team Approach for Children with Emotional Disorders: Two Case Studies." *Child & Youth Case Forum* 28, no. 2 (1998): 105–121.

Kongable, L. G., K. C. Buckwalter, and J. M. Stolley. "The Effects of Pet Therapy on the Social Behavior of Institutionalized Alzheimer's Clients." *Archives of Psychiatric Nursing* 3, no. 4 (August 1989): 191–98.

Krol, William. "Training the Combat and Operational Stress Control Dog: An Innovative Modality for Behavioral Health." *U.S. Army Medical Department Journal* (April-June 2012): 46–50.

Kruger, Katherine A., and James A. Serpell.

"Animal-Assisted Interventions in Mental Health: Definitions and Theoretical Foundations." In *Handbook on Animal-Assisted Therapy: Theoretical Foundations and Guidelines for Practice,* 2nd ed., edited by Aubrey Fine, 21–38. Amsterdam: Elsevier, 2006.

Kuhl, Gail. "Human-Sled Dog Relations: What Can We Learn from the Stories and Experiences of Mushers?" *Society and Animals* 19 (2011): 23–37. http://www.animalsandsociety.org/wp-content/uploads/2016/05/kuhl.pdf.

Labelle, Leslie J. "Considering Pet Therapy? How to Write Your Hospital's Animal Policy." The Joint Commission, July 20, 2017. https://www.jointcommission.org/considering-pet-therapy-here%E2%80%99s-how-to-write-your-hospital%E2%80%99s-animal-policy/.

Langley, Gerald, Kevin M. Nolan, Thomas W. Nolan, Clifford Norman, and Lloyd P. Provost. *The Improvement Guide: A Practical Approach to Enhancing Organizational Performance.* San Francisco: Jossey-Bass, 1996.

Langley, Gerald J., Ronald D. Moen, Kevin M. Nolan, Thomas W. Nolan, Clifford L. Norman, and Lloyd P. Provost. *The Improvement Guide: A Practical Approach to Enhancing Organizational Performance.* 2nd ed. San Francisco, CA: Jossey-Bass, 2009.

Lash, Joseph P. *Helen and Teacher: The Story of Helen Keller and Anne Sullivan Macy.* New York: Da Capo Press, 1980.

Lee, D. (1984). "Companion Animals in Institutions." In *Dynamic Relationships in Practice: Animals in the Helping Professions,* edited by Phil Arkow, 229–36. Alameda, CA: Latham Foundation, 1984.

Lefebvre, S. L., G. C. Golab, E. Christensen, L. Castrodale, K. Aureden, A. Bialachowski, N. Gumley, J. Robinson, A. Peregrine, M. Benoit, M. L. Card, L. Van Hore, and J. S. Weese. "Guidelines for Animal Assisted Interventions in Health Care Facilities." *American Journal of Infection Control* 36 (2008): 78–85. doi: 10.1016/j.ajic.2007.09.005.

Levine, G. N., K. Allen, L. T. Braun, H. E. Christian, E. Friedmann, K. A. Taubert, S. A. Thomas, D. L. Wells, and R. A. Lange. "Pet Ownership and Cardiovascular Risk: A Scientific Statement From the American Heart Association." *Circulation* 127, no. 23 (2013): 2353–63.

Levinson, Boris M. *The Animal Companion and the Emotionally Handicapped Child.* Paper presented at the Blueberry Treatment Center, Brooklyn, NY, 1979.

Levinson, Boris M. "The Dog as a 'Co-Therapist.'" *Mental Hygiene* 46 (1962): 59–65.

Levinson, Boris M. "The Future of Research into Relationships Between People and Their Animal Companions." *International Journal for the Study of Animal Problems* 3, no. 4 (1982): 283–93.

Levinson, Boris M. "Household Pets in Residential Schools: Their Therapeutic Potential." *Mental Hygiene* 52, no. 3 (July 1968): 411–14.

Levinson, Boris M. *Pet-Oriented Child Psychotherapy.* Springfield, IL: Charles C. Thomas, 1969.

Levinson, Boris M. *Pets and Human Development.* Springfield, IL: Thomas, 1972.

Levinson, Boris M. "Pets and Personality Development." *Psychological Reports* 42 (1978): 1031–38.http://scholar.google.com/scholar_lookup?title=Petsandpersonalitydevelopment&author=B..Levinson&journal=PsychologicalReports&volume=42&pages=1031-1038&publication_year=1978 doi:10.2466/pr0.1978.42.3c.1031.

Levinson, Boris M. "Pets, Child Development, and Mental Illness." *Journal of the American Veterinary Medical Association* 157, no. 11 (1970): 1759–66.

Levinson, Boris M. "Pets: A Special Technique in Child Psychotherapy." *Mental Hygiene* 48, no. 2 (April 1964): 243–48.

Levinson, Boris M. "Special Technique in Child Psychotherapy." In *Children Away from Home: A Sourcebook of Residential Treatment,* edited by James K. Whittaker and Albert E. Trieschman, 376–82. Chicago: Aldine/Atherton, 1972.

Levinson, Boris M. "The Veterinarian and Mental Hygiene." *Mental Health* 49 (1965): 320–23.

Levinson, Boris M., and Gerald P. Mallon. *Pet-Oriented Child Psychotherapy,* 2nd ed. Springfield, IL: C. C. Thomas, 1997.

Libby, Tracy J. *Reporting for Duty: True Stories of Wounded Veterans and Their Service Dogs.* Irvine, CA: Lumina Media, 2015.

Linder, Deborah E., Hannah C. Siebens, Megan K. Mueller, Debra M. Gibbs, and Lisa M. Freeman. "Animal-Assisted Interventions: A National Survey of Health and Safety Policies in Hospitals, Eldercare Facilities, and Therapy Animal Organizations." *American Journal of Infection Control* 45, no. 8 (2017): 883–87. doi:10.1016/j.ajic.2017.04.287.

Lloyd, Janice, Claire Budge, Steve La Grow, and Kevin Stafford K. "An Investigation of the Complexities of Successful and Unsuccessful Guide Dog Matching and Partnerships." *Frontiers in Veterinary Science* 3 (2016): 114. doi: 10.3389/fvets.2016.00114.

Long, Rick. "May 16, 1938 Through Buddy's Eyes." *Today in History,* May 16, 2017. https://todayinhistory.blog/2017/05/16/may-16-1938-seeing-eye-dog/.

López-Cepero Borrego, Javier, Luis Rodríguez Franco, Maria A. Perea Mediavilla, Nuria

Blanco Piñero, Arcadio Tejada Roldán, and Alfonso Blanco Picabia. "Animal-Assisted Interventions: Review of Current Status and Future Challenges." *International Journal of Psychology and Psychological Therapy* 14, no. 1 (March 2014): 85–101.

Lundqvist, Martina, Per Carlsson, Rune Sjödahl, Elvar Theodorsson, and Lars-Åke Levin. "Patient Benefit of Dog-Assisted Interventions in Health Care: A Systematic Review." *BMC Complementary and Alternative Medicine* 17, no. 1 (2017): 358. doi: 10.1186/s12906-017-1844-7.

MacClean, Evan L., and Brian Hare. "Dogs Hijack the Human Bonding Pathway." *Science* 348, no. 6232 (2015): 280–81. doi:10.1126/science.aab1200

Mallon, Gerald, Samuel B. Ross Jr., Steve Klee, and Lisa Ross. "Designing and Implementing Animal-Assisted Therapy Programs in Health and Mental Health Organizations." In *Handbook on Animal-Assisted Therapies*, 3rd ed., edited by Aubrey Fine, 135–147. San Diego, CA: Elsevier.

Mallon, Gerald P. "Preface." In *Pet-Oriented Child Psychotherapy*, 2nd ed. Springfield, IL: Charles C. Thomas, 1997.

Mallon, Gerald P. "Utilization of Animals as Therapeutic Adjuncts with Children and Youth: A Review of the Literature." *Child & Youth Care Forum* 21, no. 1 (1992): 53–67. doi:10.1007/bf00757348.

Marcus, D. A. "Complementary Medicine in Cancer Care: Adding a Therapy Dog to the Team." *Current Pain and Headache Reports* 16, no. 4 (2012): 289–91. doi:10.1007/s11916-012-0264-0.

Marcus, D. A., C. D. Bernstein, J. M. Constantin, F. A. Kunkel, P. Breuer, and R. B. Hanlon. "Animal-Assisted Therapy at an Outpatient Pain Management Clinic." *Pain Medicine* 13 (2012): 45–57. doi:10.1111/j.1526-4637.2011.01294.x

Marr, Carolyn A., Linda French, Donna Thompson, Larry Drum, Gloria Greening, Jill Mormon, Irie Henderson, and Carroll W. Hughes. "Animal-Assisted Therapy in Psychiatric Rehabilitation." *Anthrozoös* 13 (2000): 43–47.

Marston, Holloway, and Alicia Kopicki. "The Impact of Service Dogs on Posttraumatic Stress Disorder in the Veteran Population." *The Military Psychologist* 30 no. 1 (Spring 2015): 16–21. http://www.apadivisions.org/division-19/publications/newsletters/military/2015/04/service-dogs.aspx.

Mason, Margaret S., and Christine B. Hagan. "Pet-Assisted Psychotherapy." *Psychological Reports* 84, no. 3 (1999): 1235–45. doi:10.2466/pr0.1999.84.3c.1235

Masson, Jeffrey Moussaieff, and Susan McCarthy. *When Elephants Weep: The Emotional Lives of Animals.* Auckland, New Zealand: Royal New Zealand Foundation of the Blind, 2013.

Matchock, R. L. "Pet Ownership and Physical Health." *Current Opinion in Psychiatry* 28, no. 5 (2015): 386–92. doi: 10.1097/YCO.0000000000000183.

Maujean, Annick, Christopher A. Pepping, and Elizabeth Kendall. "A Systematic Review of Randomized Controlled Trials of Animal-Assisted Therapy on Psychosocial Outcomes." *Anthrozoös* 28, no. 1 (2015): 23–36.

Mayo Clinic. "Mental Health: Overcoming the Stigma of Mental Illness." Accessed May 25, 2018. https://www.mayoclinic.org/diseases-conditions/mental-illness/in-depth/mental-health/art-20046477.

McCardle, Peggy, Sandra McCune, James A. Griffin, and Valerie Maholmes (Eds.). *How Animals Affect Us: Examining the Influence of Human-Animal Interaction on Child Development and Human Health.* Washington, D.C.: American Psychological Association.

McCardle, Peggy D. *How Animals Affect Us: Examining the Influence of Human-Animal Interaction on Child Development and Human Health.* Washington, D.C.: American Psychological Association, 2011.

McCarthey, Meghan. *The Incredible Life of Balto.* New York: Knopf, 2011.

McConell, Edwina A. "Myths & Facts About Animal-Assisted Therapy." *Nursing* 32, no. 3 (March 2002): 76.

McCullough, A., A. Ruehrdanz, M. Jenkins, and R. Ganzert. "The Importance of Assessing Behavioral and Physiological Stress in Therapy Dogs." *Austin Journal of Veterinary Science & Animal Husbandry* 2, no. 1 (2015): 1008.

McCullough, Amy, Ashleigh Ruehrdanz, and Molly Jenkins. *The Use of Dogs in Hospital Settings* [HABRI Central Briefs]. Human-Animal Bond Research Institute, January 18, 2016. https://habricentral.org/resources/54871/download/hc_brief_dogsinhospitals20160115Access.pdf.

McCullough, Amy, Ashleigh Ruehrdanz, Molly A. Jenkins, Mary Jo Gilmer, Janice Olson, Anjali Pawar, Leslie Holley, et al. "Measuring the Effects of an Animal-Assisted Intervention for Pediatric Oncology Patients and Their Parents: A Multisite Randomized Controlled Trial." *Journal of Pediatric Oncology Nursing* 35, no. 3 (2017): 159–77.

McCullough, Amy, Molly A. Jenkins, Ashleigh Ruehrdanz, Mary Jo Gilmer, Janice Olson, Anjali Pawar, Leslie Holley, et al. "Physiological and Behavioral Effects of Animal-Assisted Interventions on Therapy Dogs in Pediatric Oncology Settings." *Applied Animal Behaviour Science* 200 (2018): 86–95.

McCullough, Bill. "A Letter from the Founder." *Pet Partners Interactions Magazine* (Spring 2017): 3–4. Accessed January 5, 2018. https://petpartners.org/wp-content/uploads/2014/12/PetPartners-Spring17.pdf.

McCune, Sandra, Katherine A. Kruger, James A. Griffin, Layla Esposito, Lisa S. Freund, Regina Bures, Karyl J. Hurley, and Nancy R. Gee. "Strengthening the Foundation of Human-Animal Interaction Research: Recent Developments in a Rapidly Growing Field." In *Handbook on Animal-Assisted Therapy: Foundations and Guidelines for Animal-Assisted Interventions,* 4th ed., edited by Aubrey Fine, 408–13. San Diego, CA: Academic Press, 2015.

McDonald, Lynn. *Florence Nightingale at First Hand.* London: Continuum UK, 2010.

McDonald, Lynn. "An Unscrupulous Liar? Florence Nightingale Revealed in Her Own Writings." *Times Literary Supplement,* December 8, 2000, 14–15.

McDonald, Lynn (Ed.). *The Collected Works of Florence Nightingale* (16 volumes). Waterloo: Wilfrid Laurier University Press, 2002–2013.

McDonald, Lynn (Ed.). *Florence Nightingale: An Introduction to Her Life and Family, Volume 1 of The Collected Works of Florence Nightingale.* Waterloo: Wilfrid Laurier University Press, 2002.

McKinney, M. "Why More Hospitals Are Letting Pets Visit Their Sick Owners." Vet Street, 2014. Accessed December 30, 2017. http://www.vetstreet.com/our-pet-experts/why-more-hospitals-are-letting-pets-visit-their-sickowners.

McNicholas, June, and Glyn M. Collis. "Dogs as Catalysts for Social Interaction: Robustness of the Effect." *British Journal of Psychology* 91 (2000): 61–70. doi: 10.1348/000712600161673.

McQuillen, Debby. "Pet Therapy: Initiating a Program." *Canadian Journal of Occupational Therapy* 52, no. 2 (1985): 73–76. doi:10.1177/000841748505200204.

Mellor, David J. "Moving Beyond the 'Five Freedoms' by Updating the 'Five Provisions' and Introducing Aligned 'Animal Welfare Aims.'" *Animals* 6, no. 10 (October 2016): 59.

Melson, Gail F. *Why the Wild Things Are: Animals in the Lives of Children.* Cambridge, MA: Harvard University Press, 2001.

Melson, Gail F., and Aubrey H. Fine. "Animals in the Lives of Children." In *Handbook on Animal-Assisted Therapies,* 3rd ed., edited by Aubrey Fine, 223–46. San Diego, CA: Elsevier, 2010.

Meredith, L. S., C. D. Sherbourne, S. Gaillot, L. Hansell, H. V. Ritschard, A. M. Parker, et al. *Promoting Psychological Resilience in the U.S. Military.* Santa Monica, CA: Rand Corporation, 2011.

Michalko, Rod. *The Difference That Disability Makes.* Philadelphia: Temple University Press, 2002.

Michalko, Rod. *The Two-in-One: Walking with Smokie, Walking with Blindness.* Philadelphia: Temple University Press, 1999.

Miller, Suzanne C., Cathy C. Kennedy, Dale C. Devoe, Matthew Hickey, Tracy Nelson, and Lori Kogan. "An Examination of Changes in Oxytocin Levels in Men and Women Before and After Interaction with a Bonded Dog." *Anthrozoös* 22, no. 1 (2009): 31–42. doi:10.2752/175303708x390455.

Mills, D., and S. Hall. "Animal-Assisted Interventions: Making Better Use of the Human-Animal Bond." *Veterinary Record* 174 (2014): 269–73. doi:10.1136/vr.g1929.

Mills, James T., and Arthur F. Yeager. "Definition of Animals Used in Healthcare Settings." *U.S. Army Medical Department Journal* (April-June 2012): 12–17. http://www.cs.amedd.army.mil/filedownloadpublic.aspx?docid=73e8d2aa-1a2a-467d-b6e3-e73652da8622.

"Miss Nightingale Dies Age 90." *New York Times.* Accessed April 30, 2018. https://archive.nytimes.com/www.nytimes.com/learning/general/onthisday/bday/0512.html.

Mitchell, Stephen A., and Margaret J. Black. *Freud and Beyond: A History of Modern Psychoanalytical Thought.* New York: Basic Books, 1995.

Molnar, Michael. "Of Dogs and Doggerel." *American Imago* 53, no. 3 (1996): 269–280.

Moretti, Francesca, Diana De Ronchi, Virginia Bernabei, Lucia Marchetti, Barbara Ferrari, Claudia Forlani, Francesca Negretti, Cleta Sacchetti, and Anna Rita Atti. "Pet Therapy in Elderly Patients with Mental Illness." *Psychogeriatrics* 11, no. 2 (June 2011): 125–29. doi:10.1111/j.1479-8301.2010.00329.x.

Moyer, Steve. "Dog vs. Airplane." *Humanities* 34, no. 6 (2013, November/December).

Murphy, Kathryn. "Animals in Healthcare Settings." *Nursing Made Incredibly Easy* 13, no. 6 (2015): 42–48. https://www.nursingcenter.com/cearticle?an=00152258-201511000-00010&Journal_ID=417221&Issue_ID=3218692

Murthy, Rekha, Gonzalo Bearman, Sherrill Brown, Kristina Bryant, Raymond Chinn, Angela Hewlett, B. Glenn George, et al. "Animals in Healthcare Facilities: Recommendations to Minimize Potential Risks." *Infection Control & Hospital Epidemiology* 36, no. 5 (2015): 495–516. doi:10.1017/ice.2015.15.

Muschel, I. J. "Pet Therapy with Terminal Cancer Patients." *Social Casework* 65, no. 8 (October 1984): 451–58.

Museum of Healthcare at Kingston. "Diphtheria." Accessed October 19, 2017. http://www.museumofhealthcare.ca/explore/exhibits/vaccinations/diphtheria.html.

Naderi, Sz., A. Miklósi, A. Dóka, and V. Csányi. "Co-operative Interactions Between Blind Persons and Their Dogs." *Applied Animal Behaviour Science* 74, no. 1 (2001): 59–80. http://dx.doi.org/10.1016/S0168-1591(01)00152-6.

Nagasawa, Miho, Shouhei Mitsui, Shiori En, Nobuyo Ohtani, Mitsuaki Ohta, Yasuo Sakuma, Tatsushi Onaka, Kazutaka Mogi, and Takefumi Kikusui. "Oxytocin-Gaze Positive Loop and the Coevolution of Human-Dog Bonds." *Science* 438, no. 6232 (2015): 333–36. doi:10.1126/science.1261022.

National Alliance on Mental Illness. "Stigma*free*." Accessed November 15, 2017. https://www.nami.org/stigmafree.

National Archives. *Florence Nightingale*. Accessed September 16, 2017. http://www.nationalarchives.gov.uk/education/resources/florence-nightingale/.

National Archives. Records of the Public Health Service [PHS], 1912–1968. Record Group 90. Accessed October 19, 2017. https://www.archives.gov/research/guide-fed-records/groups/090.html.

National Link Coalition, "What is the Link?" Accessed October 10, 2018. http://nationallinkcoalition.org/faqs/what-is-the-link

Natterson-Horowitz, Barbara, and Kathryn Bowers. *Zoobiquity: The Astonishing Connection Between Human and Animal Health*. New York: Random House, 2013.

Nepps, P., C. N. Stewart, and S. R. Bruckno. "Animal-Assisted Activity: Effects of a Complementary Invention Program on Psychological and Physiological Variables." *Journal of Evidence-Based Complementary & Alternative Medicine* 19, no. 3 (2014): 211–15. doi:10.1177/2156587214533570.

"New Guidance for Animal Hospital Visits Released." *Healthcare Risk Management Review*, April 3, 2015. https://www.hrmronline.com/news/new-guidance-for-animal-hospital-visits-released-751.

New York City Parks. "Central Park: Balto." Accessed October 7, 2017. https://www.nycgovparks.org/parks/central-park/monuments/75.

Newton, Robyn. *Exploring the Experiences of Living with Psychiatric Service Dogs for Veterans with Posttraumatic Stress Disorder*. Thesis, Adler School of Professional Psychology, 2014.

Ng, Zenithson, Julie Albright, Aubrey H. Fine, and Jose Peralta. "Our Ethical and Moral Responsibility: Ensuring the Welfare of Therapy Animals." In *Handbook on Animal-Assisted Therapy*, 4th ed., edited by Aubrey H. Fine, 357–76. Amsterdam: Elsevier Academic Press, 2015.

Nicholson, Jill, Susan Kemp-Wheeler, and David Griffiths. "Distress Arising from the End of a Guide Dog Partnership." *Anthrozoös* 8 (1995): 100–110. doi:10.2752/089279395787156419.

Nightingale, Florence. *Cassandra*. New York: Feminist Press, 1979.

Nightingale, Florence. "Letters of Florence Nightingale." *Yale Review* 12 (1934): 326–47.

Nightingale, Florence. *Notes on Hospitals*. London: John W. Parker & Son, 1859.

Nightingale, Florence. *Notes on Nursing*. New York: D. Appleton and Company. Accessed September 16, 2017. http://digital.library.upenn.edu/women/nightingale/nursing/nursing.html.

Nightingale Museum. *Florence Nightingale Biography*. Accessed September 14, 2017. http://www.florence-nightingale.co.uk/resources/biography/?v=7516fd43adaa.

Nilsson, Jeff, Andy Hollandbeck, and Dorothy Harrison Eustis. "The Post Article that Launched the Seeing Eye Program." *The Saturday Evening Post*, April 14, 2016. http://www.saturdayeveningpost.com/2016/04/14/history/post-perspective/post-article-launched-seeing-eye-program.html.

Nimer, Janelle, and Brad Lundahl. "Animal-Assisted Therapy: A Meta-Analysis." *Antrozoos* 20, no. 3 (2015): 225–38. https://doi.org/10.2752/089279307X224773.

"No More Dogs Needed Please." *Red Cross Magazine* 13 no. 1 (January 2018).

Nordgren, L., and G. Engstrom. "Animal-Assisted Intervention in Dementia: Effects on Quality of Life." *Clinical Nursing Research* 23 (2014): 7–19.

Norman, Jim. "Americans Rate Healthcare Providers High on Honesty, Ethics." *Gallup News*, December 19, 2016. http://news.gallup.com/poll/200057/americans-rate-health care-providers-high-honesty-ethics.aspx.

O'Callaghan, Dana M., and Cynthia K. Chandler. "An Exploratory Study of Animal-Assisted Interventions Utilized by Mental Health Professionals." *Journal of Creativity in Mental Health* 6, no. 2 (2011): 90–104. http://dx.doi.org/10.1080/15401383.2011.579862.

O'Callaghan, Dana M., and Cynthia K. Chandler. "An Exploratory Study of Animal-Assisted Interventions Utilized by Mental Health Professionals." *Journal of Creativity in Mental Health* 6, no. 2 (2011): 90–104.

Odendaal, J. S. J. "Animal-Assisted Therapy— Magic or Medicine?" *Journal of Psychosomatic Research* 49, no. 4 (2000): 275–80. doi:10.1016/s0022-3999(00)00183-5.

Odendaal, Johannes, and Roy Alec Meintjes. "Neurophysiological Correlates of Affiliative Behaviour Between Humans and Dogs." *The Veterinary Journal* 165, no. 3 (2003): 296–301.

O'Haire, Marguerite E. "Animal-Assisted Intervention for Autism Spectrum Disorder: A Systematic Literature Review." *Journal of Autism and Developmental Disorders* 43, no.7 (2013): 1606–22.

O'Haire, Marguerite E., Noemie A. Guérin, and Alison C. Kirkham. "Animal-Assisted Intervention for Trauma: A Systematic Literature Review." *Frontiers in Psychology* 6 (2015): 1121. http://doi.org/10.3389/fpsyg.2015.01121.

"One Health." UC Davis, accessed June 15, 2018. https://www.ucdavis.edu/one-health/what-is-one-health.

One Health Initiative. "About the One Health Initiative." Accessed May 5, 2018. http://onehealthinitative.com/about.php.

O'Neil, J. "Summarizing 25 Years of Research on Men's Gender Role Conflict Using the Gender Role Conflict Scale: New Research Paradigms and Clinical Implications. *The Counseling Psychologist,* 36, no. 3 (2008): 358–445.

Orlandi, Massimo, Karina Trangeled, Andrea Mambrini, Mauro Tagliani, Ada Ferrarini, Liana Zanetti, Roberta Tartarini, Paola Pacetti, and Maurizio Cantore. "Pet Therapy Effects on Oncological Day Hospital Patients Undergoing Chemotherapy Treatment." *Anticancer Research* 27, no. 6C (Nov.–Dec. 2007): 4301–03.

O'Toole, Marie T. (Ed.). *Miller-Keane Encyclopedia & Dictionary of Medicine, Nursing & Allied Health,* 7th ed. Philadelphia: Saunders, 2005.

Parenti, Lindsay, Anne Foreman, B. Jean Meade, and Oliver Wirth. "A Revised Taxonomy of Assistance Animals." *Journal of Rehabilitation Research and Development* 50, no. 6 (2013): 745–56. doi:10.1682/jrrd.2012.11.0216.

Parish-Plass, Nancy. "Animal-Assisted Therapy with Children Suffering from Insecure Attachment Due to Abuse and Neglect: A Method to Lower the Risk of Intergenerational Transmission of Abuse?" *Clinical Child Psychology and Psychiatry* 13 (2008): 7–30.

Parran, Thomas, and the Alaska Health Survey Team. *Alaska's Health: A Survey Report.* 1954. Accessed October 19, 2017. http://dhss.alaska. gov/commissioner/documents/pdf/parran_report.pdf.

Parshall, Debra Phillips. "Research and Reflection: Animal-Assisted Therapy in Mental Health Settings." *Counseling and Values* 48, no. 1 (2003): 47–56. doi:10.1002/j.2161-007x. 2003.tb00274.x.

Parslow, R. A., A. F. Jorm, H. Christensen, B. Rodgers, and P. Jacomb. "Pet Ownership and Health in Older Adults: Findings from a Survey of 2,551 Community-Based Australians Aged 60–64." *Gerontology* 51, no. 1 (2005): pp. 40–47.

Peacock, J., A. Chur-Hansen, and H. Winefield. "Mental Health Implications of Human Attachment to Companion Animals." *Journal of Clinical Psychology,* 68 (2012): 292–303.

The Pet Effect. "The Science." Accessed January 5, 2018. https://thepeteffect.org/the-science.

Pet Partners. "About Us." Accessed May 24, 2018. https://petpartners.org/about-us/who-we-are/

Pet Partners. "Benefits of the Human-Animal Bond." Accessed January 5, 2018. https://petpartners.org/learn/benefits-human-animal-bond/?_ga=2.267938638.17850746.

Pet Partners. "Financial Information." Accessed June 19, 2018. https://petpartners.org/about-us/financial-information/

Pet Partners. "In 2017, About 3 Million Visits Will Be Made Across all 50 states." *Interactions Magazine* (Spring 2017): 2. https://petpartners.org/wp-content/uploads/2014/12/PetPartners-Spring17.pdf.

Pet Partners. "Library: General Health Benefits of Animals." Last modified January 24, 2013. http://www.petpartners.org/page.aspx?pid=333

Pet Partners. "Major Rumayor and Lexy: Serving our Country at Fort Bragg." *Pet Partners Interactions Magazine* (Winter 2015): 2–3. https://petpartners.org/wp-content/uploads/2015/05/Pet-Partners-Interactions-Winter-2015.pdf.

Pet Partners. "Pet Partners and the Importance of National Standards." *Interactions Magazine* (Spring 2017): 9. https://petpartners.org/wp-content/uploads/2014/12/PetPartners-Spring17.pdf.

Pet Partners. *Pet Partners Annual Report 2016.* Accessed January 5, 2018.

Pet Partners. "The Pet Partners Story." Accessed January 5, 2018. https://petpartners.org/about-us/petpartners-story/.

Pet Partners. *Pet Partners Therapy Animal Team Program Guide* [Ebook]. Bellevue: Pet Partners, 2018.

Pet Partners. "A Researcher Remembers." *Interactions Magazine* (Spring 2017): 6. https:

//petpartners.org/wp-content/uploads/2014/12/PetPartners-Spring17.pdf.

Pet Partners. *Standards of Practice in Animal Intervention* [Ebook]. Bellevue: Pet Partners, 2018.

Pet Partners. "Terminology." Accessed December 30, 2017. https://petpartners.org/learn/terminology/.

Pet Partners. "Volunteer Policies and Procedures." Accessed January 5, 2018. https://petpartners.org/volunteer/our-therapy-animal-program/volunteer-policies-procedures/.

Pet Partners Greater Dallas. "What We Do." Accessed May 24, 2018. http://petpartnersgreaterdallas.com/

Phillips, Adam. *Becoming Freud: The Making of a Psychoanalyst.* New Haven, CT: Yale University Press, 2014.

Phillips, Adam. "Introduction." In *Tribute to Freud.* New York: New Directions Books, 2012.

Pichot, Teri. *Animal-Assisted Brief Therapy: A Solution-Focused Approach.* New York: Routledge, 2012.

Polheber, J. P., and R. L. Matchock. "The Presence of a Dog Attenuates Cortisol and Heart Rate in the Trier Social Stress Test Compared to Human Friends." *Journal of Behavioral Medicine* 37, no. 2 (2014): 860–67.

Pollock, Richard A. "Triage and Management of the Injured in World War I: The Diuturnity of Antoine De Page and a Belgian Colleague." *Craniomaxillofacial Trauma and Reconstruction* 1 (2008): 63–70. doi:10.1055/s-0028-1098965.

Pols, Hans, and Stephanie Oak. "War and Military Mental Health: The US Psychiatric Response in the 20th Century." *American Journal of Public Health* 97, no. 12 (2007): 2132–42.

Pomerance, Diane. "Pets and Spirituality." *Ezine Articles,* May 13, 2008. http://ezinearticles.com/?Pets-And-Spirituality&id=1174561.

Pop, Denisa Ana, Alina Simona Rusu, Vlad Pop-Vancea, Ionel Papuc, Radu Contantinescu, and Vioara Miresan. "Physiological Effects of Human-Animal Positive Interaction in Dogs—Review of the Literature." *Bulletin of University of Agricultural Sciences and Veterinary Medicine Cluj-Napoca Animal Science and Biotechnologies* 71, no. 2 (2014): 102–10. doi:10.15835/buasvmcn-asb:10398.

Prasad, Mini. *Caesar the Anzac dog.* Auckland War Memorial Museum—Tāmaki Paenga Hira. First published November 29, 2016, Updated April 26, 2018. Accessed June 30, 2018. www.aucklandmuseum.com/war-memorial/online-cenotaph/features/caesar-the-anzac-dog

Putnam, Peter Brick. *Love in the Lead,* 2nd ed.

Lanham, MD: University Press of America, 1997.

Rabinowitz, Peter. "Training Health Care Providers About the Human-Animal Bond." Presentation at The Professionalizing the Passion Pet Partners Conference, September 2017. https://petpartners.org/wp-content/uploads/2017/01/Peter-Rabinowitz_conf2017.pdf.

Raina, P., D. Waltner-Toews, B. Bonnett, C. Woodward, and T. Abernathy. "Influence of Companion Animals on the Physical and Psychological Health of Older People: An Analysis of a One-Year Longitudinal Study." *Journal of the American Geriatrics Society* 47, no. 3 (1999): 323–29.

RAND Corporation. "One in Five Iraq and Afghanistan Veterans Suffer from PTSD and Major Depression." Press release, April 17, 2008. www.rand.org/news/press/2008/04/17.

Rankin, Joy Lisi. "Florence Nightingale: Of Myths and Maths." *The New Inquiry,* February 16, 2017. https://thenewinquiry.com/blog/florence-nightingale-of-myths-and-maths/.

"Red Cross Dogs." *The Literary Digest,* March 24, 1917, pp. 811–2. http://www.unz.org/Pub/LiteraryDigest-1917mar24-00811?View=PDF

Regier, Darrel A., William E. Narrow, Donald S. Rae, Ronald W. Manderscheid, Ben Z. Locke, and Frederick K. Goodwin. "The De Facto US Mental and Addictive Disorders Service System. Epidemiologic Catchment Area Prospective 1-Year Prevalence Rates of Disorders and Services." *Archives of General Psychiatry* 50, no. 2 (1993): 85–94. doi:10.1001/archpsyc.1993.01820140007001.

Reiser, L. W. "Topsy—Living and Dying: A Footnote to History." *The Psychoanalytic Quarterly* 56, no. 4 (1987): 667–88.

Richardson, Edwin Hautenville. *British War Dogs: Their Training and Psychology.* London: S. Skeffington and Son Ltd., 1920.

Richardson, Edwin Hautenville. *Forty Years with Dogs.* London: Hutchinson and Co., 1919. https://archive.org/details/in.ernet.dli.2015.221023.

Ricker, Elizabeth M. *Seppala: Alaska Sled Dog Driver.* Boston: Little-Brown and Company, 1930.

Rights of Blind and Physically Disabled Persons, Stat. D.C. Code Ann. § 7-1009 (2012).

Ritchie, Elspeth C., and Robinette J. Amaker. "Canine-Assisted Therapy in Military Medicine. The Early Years." *U.S. Army Medical Department Journal* 2 (2012): 5–7. http://www.cs.amedd.army.mil/filedownloadpublic.aspx?docid=73e8d2aa-1a2a-467d-b6e3-e73652da8622.

Ritchie, Elspeth C., David Benedek, Ricky Malone, and Rosemary Carr-Malone. "Psychiatry and the Military: An Update." *Psychiatric Clinics of North America* 29 (2006): 695–707. doi: http://dx.doi.org/10.1016/j.psc.2006.04. 008.

Rocco, Lucio. *The Extraordinary Work of Collies in the First World War*. Venegone Inferiore, Italy: Società Italiana Collie, not dated. http://www.colliesinitaly.it/files/book.pdf.

Rogers, Carl. "Psychotherapy Today or Where Do We Go from Here?" *American Journal of Psychotherapy* 17 (1963): 5–17.

Rogers, Everett. New York: Simon & Schuster, 2013.

Rosa, Kristi. "Battling Canine Post-Traumatic Stress Disorder." *American Veterinarian*, August 16, 2016. http://www.american veterinarian.com/news/battling-canine-posttraumatic-stress-disorder.

Rosenfeld, Gavriel D. "Counterfactual Canines: How Would History Have Been Different Without Dogs?" Blog, January 8, 2014. http://thecounterfactualhistoryreview. blogspot.com/search?q=dogs.

Rossbach, K. A., and J. P. Wilson. "Does a Dog's Presence Make a Person Appear More Likable? Two Studies." *Anthrozoös* 5, no. 1 (1992): 40–51.

Rossetti, Jeanette, Susanne Defabilis, and Camille Belpedio. "Behavioral Health Staff's Perceptions of Pet-Assisted Therapy." *Journal of Psychosocial Nursing and Mental Health Services* 46, no. 9 (2008): 28–33. doi:10.3928/ 02793695-20080901-13.

Rowell, M. C. (1990). "Creature Comfort: Animals as Therapists." *California Pharmacist*, 37 (10), 37–40.

Rubenstein, David A., Mustapha Debboun, and Richard Burton. "Perspectives." *U.S. Army Medical Department Journal* (2012, Apr-Jun): 1–4. http://www.cs.amedd.army. mil/filedownloadpublic.aspx?docid=73e 8d2aa-1a2a-467d-b6e3-e73652da8622.

Rugaas, Turid. *On Talking Terms with Dogs: Calming Signals*. 2nd ed. Wenatchee, WA: Dogwise Publishing, 2006.

Rumayor, Christine B., and Amy M. Thrasher. "Reflections on Recent Research into Animal-Assisted Interventions in the Military and Beyond." *Current Psychiatry Reports* 19, no. 12 (2017):110. doi: 10.1007/s11920-017-0861-z.

Sachs-Ericsson, N., N. K. Hansen, and S. Fitzgerald. "Benefits of Assistance Dogs: A Review." *Rehabilitation Psychology* 47 (2002): 251–77.

Salisbury, Gay, and Laney Salisbury. *The Cruelest Miles: The Heroic Story of Dogs and Men in a Race Against an Epidemic*. New York: W. W. Norton & Company, 2005.

Sanders, Clinton R. "The Impact of Guide Dogs on the Identity of People with Visual

Impairments." *Anthrozoös* 13 (2000): 131–9. doi: 10.2752/089279300786999815.

Scheindlin, Stanley. "The Drug that Launched a Thousand Sleds." *Molecular Interventions* 8, no. 4 (2008): 152–8. doi:10.1124/mi.8.4.2.

Schilp, Jill. "Dog Barks Amen as Garland Church Blesses Certified Therapy Animals Including a Local Pig." *Dallas Morning News*, March 25, 2015. https://www.dallas news.com/life/pets/2015/03/25/dog-barks-amen-as-garland-church-blesses-certified-therapy-animals-including-a-local-pig

Schilp, Jill. "Is Your Dog's Gaze the Look of Love?" *Dallas Morning News*, April 20, 2015. https://www.dallasnews.com/life/pets/2015/ 04/20/is-your-dogs-gaze-the-look-of-love-new-study-says-the-eyes-may-have-it.

Schilp, Jill. "Rescued Husky Returns Favor in Texas." *Pet Partners Interactions Magazine* (Winter 2016): 6–7. https://petpartners.org/ wp-content/uploads/2014/12/PetPartners-Magazine-Winter-2016.pdf

Schubert, Jan. "Dogs and Human Health/Mental Health: From the Pleasure of Their Company to the Benefits of Their Assistance." *U.S. Army Medical Department Journal* (April-June 2012): 21–9. http://www.cs.amedd.army. mil/filedownloadpublic.aspx?docid= 73e8d2aa-1a2a-467d-b6e3-e73652da8622.

Scovil, Elizabeth Robinson. "The Love Story of Florence Nightingale." *American Journal of Nursing* 17 (1916): 209–12.

Seal, K. H., S. Maguen, B. Cohen, K. S. Gima, T. J. Metzler, L. Ren, et al. (2010). "VA Mental Health Services Utilization in Iraq and Afghanistan Veterans in the First Year of Receiving New Mental Health Diagnoses." *Journal of Traumatic Stress* 23 (2010): 5–16.

Searles, Harold F. *The Nonhuman Environment: In Normal Development and Schizophrenia*. New York: International University Press, 1960.

The Seeing Eye. "About Vision Loss." Accessed May 22, 2018. http://www.seeingeye.org/ knowledge-center/about-vision-loss.html.

The Seeing Eye. *Annual Report 2016*. http:// www.seeingeye.org/knowledge-center/ publications/.

The Seeing Eye. "By the Numbers." 2017. http:// www.seeingeye.org/assets/pdfs/the-seeing-eye-by-the-numbers.pdf.

The Seeing Eye. "Frequently Asked Questions." Accessed June 20, 2018. http://www.seeing eye.org/about-us/faq.html.

The Seeing Eye. "History." Accessed May 22, 2018. http://www.seeingeye.org/about-us/ history.html.

Sehulster, Lynne, and Raymond Y. W. Chinn. "Guidelines for Environmental Infection Control in Health-Care Facilities. Recommendations of CDC and the Healthcare Infection Control Practices Advisory Committee (HICPAC)." *MMWR. Recommendations and Reports: Morbidity and Mortality Weekly Report* 52, no. RR-10 (June 6, 2003): 1–42.

Selanders, Louise C., and Patrick C. Crane. "The Voice of Florence Nightingale on Advocacy." *Online Journal of Issues in Nursing* 17 (January 2002): Manuscript 1. http://www.nursingworld.org/MainMenuCategories/ANAMarketplace/ANAPeriodicals/OJIN/TableofContents/Vol-17-2012/No1-Jan-2012/Florence-Nightingale-on-Advocacy.html.

Serpell, James A. "Animal Companions and Human Well-Being: An Historical Exploration of the Value of Human-Animal Relationships." In *Handbook on Animal-Assisted Therapies*, 2nd ed., edited by Aubrey Fine, 3–19. San Diego: Academic Press, 2006.

Serpell, James A. "Animal Companions and Human Well-Being: An Historical Exploration of the Value of Human-Animal Relationships." In *Handbook of Animal-Assisted Therapy: Theoretical Foundations and Guidelines for Practice,* edited by Aubrey Fine. San Diego: Academic Press, 2000.

Serpell, James A. "Animal-Assisted Interventions in Historical Perspective." In *Handbook on Animal-Assisted Therapy: Theoretical Foundations and Guidelines for Practice,* 3rd ed., edited by Aubrey Fine, 17–32. New York: Elsevier, 2010.

Serpell, James A. "Anthropomorphism and Anthropomorphic Selection—Beyond the 'Cute Response.'" *Society and Animals* 11 (2003): 83–100.

Serpell, James A. "Beneficial Effects of Pet Ownership on Some Aspects of Human Health and Behaviour." *Journal of the Royal Society of Medicine* 84 (1991): 717–20.

Serpell, James A., R. Coppinger, A. H. Fine, and J. M. Peralta. "Welfare Considerations in Therapy and Assistance Animals." In *Handbook on Animal-Assisted Therapies*, 3rd ed., edited by Aubrey Fine. San Diego: Academic Press, 2010.

Serpell, James A., Sandra McCune, Nancy Gee, and James A. Griffin. "Current Challenges to Research on Animal-Assisted Interventions." *Applied Developmental Science* 21, no. 3 (2017): pages 223–233.

Seward Park Conservatory. "Togo." Accessed October 7, 2017. https://www.sewardpark conservancy.org/present/.

Sharkin, B. S., and D. Knox. "Pet Loss: Issues and Implications for the Psychologist." *Professional Psychology: Research and Practice* 34, no. 4 (2003): 414–21.

Shiloh, Shoshana, Gal Sorek, and Joseph Terkel. "Reduction of State-Anxiety by Petting Animals in a Controlled Laboratory Experiment." *Anxiety, Stress & Coping* 16, no. 4 (2003): 387–95. doi:10.1080/10615800310000 91582.

Showalter, Allan. "Freud's Damn Dog and Other Curious Tales of Being Analyzed by Freud." Blog, May 19, 2016. http://allanshowalter.com/2016/05/19/freud-damn-dog-roy-grinker-analyzed-sigmund-freud/

Small, Hugh. *Florence Nightingale: Avenging Angel.* New York: St. Martin's, 1998.

Smith, Cecil Woodham. *Florence Nightingale 1820–1910.* London: Forgotten Books, 2017 (originally published in 1910).

Smith, F. B. *Florence Nightingale: Reputation and Power.* New York: Palgrave Macmillan, 1982.

Smith-Forbes, Enrique, Cecilia Najera, and David Hawkins. "Combat Operational Stress Control in Iraq and Afghanistan: Army Occupational Therapy." *Military Medicine* 179 (2014): 279–284. https://doi.org/10.7205/MILMED-D-13-00452.

Snipelisky, David, and M. Caroline Burton. "Canine-Assisted Therapy in the Inpatient Setting." *Southern Medical Journal* 107, no. 4 (2014): 265–73. doi:10.1097/smj.00000000 00000090.

Souter, Megan A., and Michelle D. Miller. "Do Animal-Assisted Activities Effectively Treat Depression? A Meta-Analysis." *Anthrozoös* 20, no. 2 (2007): 167–80. doi:10.2752/175303 707x207954.

Stallones, L., M. B. Marx, T. F. Garrity, and T. P. Johnson. "Pet Ownership and Attachment in Relation to the Health of U.S. Adults, 21 to 64 Years of Age." *Anthrozoös* 4, no. 2 (1990): 100–12.

Standiford, Natalie. *The Bravest Dog Ever: The True Story of Balto.* New York: Random House, 1989.

Stapleton, Mary, and Rick Parente. "Effectiveness of Animal-Assisted Therapy after Brain Injury: A Bridge to Improved Outcomes in CRT." *NeuroRehabilitation* 39, no. 1 (2016): 135–40.

Stark, Myra. "Introduction." In *Cassandra,* by Florence Nightingale, 11–15. New York: Feminist Press, 1979.

Stoeckel, Luke E., Lori S. Palley, Randy L. Gollub, Steven M. Niemi, and Anne Eden Evins. "Patterns of Brain Activation when Mothers View Their Own Child and Dog: An fMRI Study." *PLoS One* 9, no. 10 (2014). doi:10.1371/journal.pone.0107205.

Stokes, E. D. "The Race for Life." *Public Health Reports* 11 (1996, May/June): 272–5. https://www.ncbi.nlm.nih.gov/pmc/articles/PMC1381772/pdf/pubhealthrep00048-0090.pdf.

Strachey, Lytton. *Eminent Victorians*. London: Chatto & Windus, 1918.

Strand, Elizabeth B. "Interparental Conflict and Youth Maladjustment: The Buffering Effects of Pets." *Stress, Trauma, and Crisis* 7, no. 3 (2004): 151–68.

Struckus, Joseph E. "Pet-Facilitated Therapy and the Elderly Client." In *Handbook of Clinical Behavior Therapy with the Elderly Client*, edited by P. A. Wisocki, 403–19. New York: Plenum Press, 1991.

"Stubby of A.E.F. Enters Valhalla: Tramp Dog of No Pedigree Took Part in the Big Parade in France." *New York Times*, April 4, 1926.

Stull, J. W., and K. B. Stevenson. "Zoonotic Disease Risks for Immunocompromised and Other High-Risk Clients and Staff: Promoting Safe Pet Ownership and Contact." *Veterinary Clinics of North America: Small Animal Practice* 45, no. 2 (2015): 377–92.

Stull, J. W., C. C. Hoffman, and T. Landers. "Health Benefits and Risks of Pets in Nursing Homes: A Survey of Facilities in Ohio." *Journal of Gerontological Nursing* 44, no. 5 (2018): 39–45. doi: 10.3928/00989134-20180 322-02.

Swanbeck, Steve. *Images of America: The Seeing Eye*. Charleston, SC: Arcadia Publishing, 2002.

Tabers Medical Dictionary Online. "Triage." Accessed May 10, 2018. https://www.tabers. com/tabersonline/view/Tabers-Dictionary/ 735812/all/triage?q=triage.

Teal, L. "Pet Partners Help with the Healing Process." *Interactions* 19, no. 4 (2002), 3–5.

Tedeschi, Philip. "The New Work of Intervention and Assistance Dogs: Beyond the Five Freedoms." Keynote Address Presented at the Assistance Dogs International Conference, Denver, Colorado, September 2014.

Tedeschi, Philip, Aubrey H. Fine, and Jana I. Helgeson. "Assistance Animals: Their Evolving Role in Psychiatric Service Applications." In *Handbook on Animal-Assisted Therapy: Theoretical Foundations and Guidelines for Practice*, 3rd ed., edited by Aubrey Fine, 421–38. New York: Elsevier, 2010.

Texas Health Resources. "Some Hospital Volunteers are a Breed Apart: Canine Ambassadors Active at 10 Texas Health Facilities." April 17, 2018. https://www.texashealth.org/ news/some-hospital-volunteers-are-a-breed-apart.

Texas Husky Rescue. Bellin Bellin Facebook page. Accessed December 10, 2017. https:// www.facebook.com/teambellin/

Therapy Dogs International. Home page. Accessed June 15, 2018. https://www.tdi-dog. org/default.aspx.

Thompson, John Gilbert, and Inez Bigwood.

Lest We Forget: World War Stories. Boston: Silver, Burdett and Company, 1918.

Tielsch, Anna, and May Jo Gilmer. "The Role and Impact of Animals with Pediatric Patients." *Pediatric Nursing* 41, no. 2 (March-April 2015): 65–69.

Timmons, Richard, Aubrey H. Fine, and Richard Meadows. "The Role of the Veterinary Family Practitioner in AAT and AAA programs." In *Handbook on Animal-Assisted Therapies*, 3rd ed., edited by Aubrey Fine, 505–18. San Diego: Academic Press, 2010.

Tooley, Sarah. *Life of Florence Nightingale*. London: Cassell, 1910.

Treaster, Joseph. "Elliott Humphrey 92 Pioneered in Tutoring of Guide Dogs in US" (Obituary). *The New York Times*, June 11, 1981.

Trembath, Felicia. *Practitioner Attitudes and Beliefs Regarding the Roles Animals Play in Human Health*. HABRI Central Briefs, December 19, 2014. Accessed January 6, 2018. https://habricentral.org/resources/44272/do wnload/HABRICentralBriefsPractitioner-Attitudes.pdf

Turner, D. C. The role of ethology in the field of human-animal relations and animal assisted therapy. In *Handbook on Animal-Assisted Therapies*, 2nd ed., edited by Aubrey Fine, 547–55. Amsterdam: Elsevier, 2006.

Tuttle, Dean, and Naomi Tuttle. "Morris Frank." In *Hall of Fame: Leaders and Legends of the Blindness Field*. Louisville, KY: American Printing House for the Blind, 2010. http:// www.aph.org/hall/inductees/frank/.

Underhill, Evelyn. *Practical Mysticism: A Little Book for Normal People*. New York: E. P. Dutton and Co., 1943.

Ungermann, Kenneth. *The Race to Nome*. New York: Harper and Row, 1963.

Urbanski, B. L., and M. Lazenby. "Distress Among Hospitalized Pediatric Cancer Patients Modified by Pet-Therapy Intervention to Improve Quality of Life." *Journal of Pediatric Oncology Nursing* 29, no. 5 (2012): 272–82. doi:10.1177/1043454212455697.

U.S. Army. "Careers & Jobs: Occupational Therapist (65A)." Accessed November 15, 2017. https://www.goarmy.com/careers-and-jobs/ amedd-categories/medical-specialist-corps-jobs/occupational-therapist.html.

U.S. Department of Justice, Civil Rights Division. "ADA Requirements: Service Animals." July 2011. https://www.ada.gov/service _animals_2010.pdf.

U.S. Department of Justice, Civil Rights Division, Disability Section. "Frequently Asked Questions About Service Animals and the ADA." Accessed April 25, 2018. https://www. ada.gov/regs2010/service_animal_qa.html.

U.S. Department of Veterans Affairs. "Dogs and PTSD." April 29, 2014. http://www.ptsd. va.gov/PTSD/public/treatment/cope/dogs_ and_ptsd.asp.

U.S. War Dogs Association. "World War I." Accessed June 20, 2018. http://www.uswardogs. org/war-dog-history/world-war-1/

Uvnä-Moberg, Kerstin, Linda Handlin, and Maria Petersson. "Self-Soothing Behaviors with Particular Reference to Oxytocin Release Induced by Non-Noxious Sensory Stimulation." *Frontiers in Psychology* 5 (May 2014): 1529. doi:10.3389/fpsyg.2014.01529.

Vacha, John. "Cleveland Saves Balto." *Timeline: A Publication of the Ohio Historical Society* 22, no. 1 (2005, January/March): 54–69.

Vanderbilt University. "Through Buddy's Eyes." *Vanderbilt Magazine,* December 6, 2010. https://news.vanderbilt.edu/vanderbilt-magazine/through-buddys-eyes/.

VanFleet, Risë, and Tracie Faa-Thompson. *Animal-Assisted Play Therapy.* Sarasota, FL: Professional Resource Press, 2017.

VanFleet, Risë, Aubrey H. Fine, Dana O'Callaghan, Teal Mackintosh, and Julia Gimeno. 2015. "Application of Animal-Assisted Interventions in Professional Settings." In *Handbook on Animal-Assisted Therapy,* 4th ed., edited by Aubrey H. Fine, 157–77. Amsterdam: Elsevier/Academic Press, 2015.

Vaughan, C. A., T. L. Schell, T. Tanielian, L. H. Jaycox, and G. N. Marshall. "Prevalence of Mental Health Problems Among Iraq and Afghanistan Veterans Who Have and Have Not Received VA Services." *Psychiatric Services* 65, no. 6 (2014): 833–35.

Voelker, R. "Puppy Love Can Be Therapeutic, Too." *JAMA: The Journal of the American Medical Association* 274, no. 24 (1995): 1897–1899. doi:10.1001/jama.274.24.1897.

Walsh, Froma. "Human-Animal Bonds I: The Relational Significance of Companion Animals." *Family Process* 48, no. 4 (2009): 462–480. doi: 10.1111/j.1545-5300.2009.01296.x.

Walsh, Froma. "Human-Animal Bonds II: The Role of Pets in Family Systems and Family Therapy." *Family Process* 48, no. 4 (2009): 481–499. doi:10.1111/j.1545-5300.2009.01297.x

Walter-Toews, D. "Zoonotic Disease Concerns in Animal Assisted Therapy and Animal Visitation Programs." *Canadian Veterinary Journal* 34 (1993): 549–51.

Walters Esteves, Stephanie, and Trevor Stokes. "Social Effects of a Dog's Presence on Children with Disabilities." *Anthrozoös* 21, no. 1 (2008): 5–15.

Watkins, Kathleen L. "Policy Initiatives for the Use of Canines in Military Medicine." *U.S. Army Medical Department Journal* (2012, Apr-Jun): 8–11. http://www.cs.amedd.army.

mil/filedownloadpublic.aspx?docid= 73e8d2aa-1a2a-467d-b6e3-e73652da8622. Accessed November 15, 2017.

Welch, Curtis. "The Diphtheria Epidemic at Nome." *Journal of the American Medical Association* 84 (1925): 1290–91. doi:10.1001/ jama.1925.02660430048031.

White, Jennifer H., Martina Quinn, Sheila Garland, Dale Dirkse, Patricia Wiebe, Madeline Hermann, and Linda E. Carlson. "Animal-Assisted Therapy and Counseling Support for Women With Breast Cancer: An Exploration of Patient's Perceptions." *Integrative Cancer Therapies* 14, no. 5 (2015): 460–67. doi: 10.1177/1534735415580678.

Whitmarsh, L. "The Benefits of Guide Dog Ownership." *Visual Impairment Research* 7 (2005): 27–42. http://dx.doi.org/10.1080/ 13882350590956439.

Wilkes, C. N., T. K. Shalko, and M. Trahan. "Pet Therapy: Implications for Good Health." *Health Education* 20 (1989): 6–9.

Williams, David. "From the Medical Perspective." *Pet Partners Interactions Magazine* (Spring 2017), 8–9. Accessed January 5, 2018. https://petpartners.org/wp-content/uploads/2014/12/PetPartners-Spring17.pdf.

Wilson, Cindy C., and Sandra B. Barker. "Challenges in Designing Human-Animal Interaction Research." *American Behavioral Scientist* 47, no. 1 (2003): 16–28. doi:10.1177/000 2764203255208.

Wilson, Edward O. *Biophilia.* Cambridge: Harvard University Press, 1984.

Wilson, W. H. "The Serum Dash to Nome, 1925: The Making of Alaskan Heroes." *Alaska Journal* 16 (1986): 250–59.

Wood, Emily, Sally Ohlsen, Jennifer Thompson, Joe Hulin, and Louise Knowles. "The Feasibility of Brief Dog-Assisted Therapy on University Students' Stress Levels: The PAWS Study." *Journal of Mental Health* 27, no. 3 (2017): 263–68. doi:10.1080/09638237. 2017.1385737.

Wood, Lisa, Billie Giles-Corti, and Max Bulsara. "The Pet Connection: Pets as a Conduit for Social Capital?" *Social Science & Medicine* 61, no. 6 (2005): 1159–173. doi:10.1016/j. socscimed.2005.01.017.

World Organization for Animal Health. "Animal Welfare." Accessed January 5, 2018. http://www.oie.int/en/animal-welfare/ animal-welfare-at-a-glance/.

World Organization for Animal Health. "Recognition of Animal Health Status," May 20, 1999. http://www.oie.int/en/about-us/key-texts/basic-texts/recognition-of-animal-health-status/.

Wright, Andy. "In Victorian England, a Sheep Wasn't Just a Sheep." *Modern Farmer,* December 10, 2013. https://modernfarmer.com/tag/victorian-era/.

Wu, A. S., R. Niedra, L. Pendergast, and B. W. McCrindle. "Acceptability and Impact of Pet Visitation on a Pediatric Cardiology Inpatient Unit." *Journal of Pediatric Nursing* 17, no. 5 (2002): 354–362. doi:10.1053/jpdn.2002.127173.

Wynne, William A. *Yorkie Doodle Dandy: A Memoir.* Rocky River: Lakefront Publishers, 2013.

Yamamoto, M., M. T. Lopez, and L. A. Hart. "Registrations of Assistance Dogs in California for Identification Tags: 1999–2012." *PLoS One* 10, no. 8 (2015):e0132820. doi:10.1371/journal.pone.0132820.

Yamauchi, Terry, and Esther Pipkin. "Six Years' Experience with Animal-Assisted Therapy in a Children's Hospital: Is There Patient Risk?" *American Journal of Infection Control* 36, no. 5 (2008). doi:10.1016/j.ajic.2008.04.132.

Yarborough, Bobbi Jo H., Ashli A. Owen-Smith, Scott P. Stumbo, Micah T. Yarborough, Nancy A. Perrin, and Carla A. Green. "An Observational Study of Service Dogs for Veterans with Posttraumatic Stress Disorder." *Psychiatry Services* 68 (2017): 730–4. https://doi.org/10.1176/appi.ps.201500383.

Yeager, A. F., and J. Irwin. "Rehabilitative Canine Interactions at the Walter Reed National Military Medical Center." *U.S. Army Medical Department Journal* 2 (2012): 57–60.

Yount, Rick, Elspeth C. Ritchie, Matthew St. Laurent, Perry Chumley, and Meg D. Olmert. "The Role of Service Dog Training in the Treatment of Combat-Related PTSD." *Psychiatric Annals* 43 (2013): 292–95. doi: 10.3928/00485713-20130605-11.

Index

Numbers in **bold italics** indicate pages with illustrations